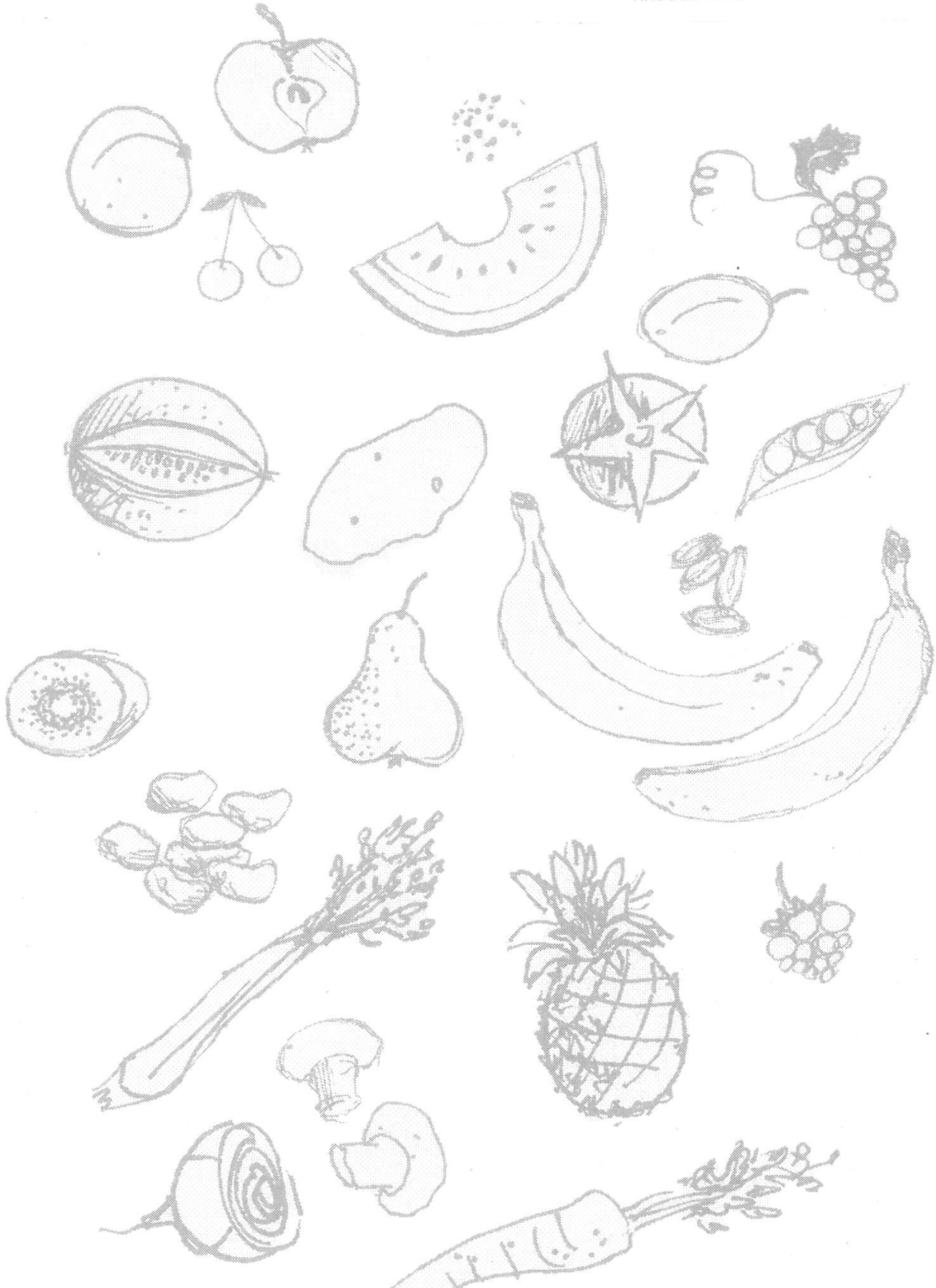

This book is intended as a reference volume only, not as a medical manual. Nothing written in this book should be viewed as a substitute for competent medical care. The information given here is designed to help you make more informed decisions about your health.
It is not intended as a substitute for any treatment that may have been prescribed by your doctor. If you suspect that you have a medical problem, we urge you to seek competent medical help.

Copyright © Anna I. Jäger

All rights reserved.
First Edition February, 2015

ISBN-13: 978-1508711490
ISBN-10: 1508711496

Reverse Diabetes Naturally

A Guide to Effectively Lower Your Blood Sugar Without Drugs by Following the Right Diet

Based on Scientific Research

Anna I. Jäger

Table of Contents

Introduction 7
    Symptoms of high blood sugar 10

1| Diabetes and Your Body: The Good, Bad, and Evil 12

2| Why High Fat Diets Cause Diabetes 16

3| Basics 20
    Eat Plenty of Starches! 21

4| Cutting Out the Evil 25

5| Building up Your Army of Superfoods 29
    The Super Foods 31
        Sweet Potato 31
        Potato 31
        Beans 31
        Corn 32
        Rice 32
        Kale 32
        Beet Greens 32
        Lamb's Quarters Plant 33
        Bok Choy 33
        Salads 33

6| Meal Planning for Low-Fat Super Meals 35

7| Doctor Visits & Reversing Diabetes 40

8| Fitness and Your Superhero Sidekick 42

9| Water – the King of all Superheroes 44

10| Blood Sugar Monitoring and Journals 46

11| Seeing the Reversal of Diabetes	49
12| Vegan Recipes	52
Breakfast	53
1| Blueberry Pancakes	54
2| French Toast	56
3| Cinnamon Berry Oatmeal	58
4| Spicy Southern Grits	60
5| Blueberry Muffins	62
6| Breakfast Cookies	64
7| Breakfast Tortillas	66
Lunch	68
1| Kale, Lemon & Cilantro Sandwich	69
2| Pesto Pasta	71
3| Black Bean Tacos	73
4| Black Beans and Rice	75
5| Mac n' Cheese	77
6| Black Bean Veggie Burger	79
7| Tomato Soup	82
Dinner	84
1| Black Bean Wrap	85
2| Quinoa Teriyaki	87
3| Shepard's Pie	89
4| Vegetable Pasta	91
5| Lasagna Rolls	93
6| Tortilla Casserole	95
7| Chickpea Chili	97
Snacks	99
1| Vanilla Chia Pudding	100
2| Baked Sweet Potato Chips	102
Final Thoughts	104
More groundbreaking studies	107
NEW: Your Body, Your Friend	108
Famous Dishes Made VEGAN!	109
Disclaimer	110
Copyright & Legal Information	110

"Type 2 diabetes is **not** a disease.
Type 2 diabetes is an adaptation.
It's a survival adaptation that the body takes."[1]
~ John McDougall, M.D.

"A low-fat vegan diet improves glycemic
control and cardiovascular risk factors in a randomized clinical trial
in individuals with type 2 diabetes."[2]

"A low-fat vegan diet and a conventional diabetes diet
in the treatment of type 2 diabetes: a randomized, controlled,
74-wk clinical trial."[3]

Meat—any meat—costs lives.
"It promotes intolerable suffering and disease—not only among animals,
but also for many Americans by raising their risk of heart disease,
diabetes, breast cancer, and early death."
~ Neal Barnard, M.D.

---

[1] HIGHLIGHTS: Dr. McDougall's Dietary Therapy: An Online Course for Reversing Common Diseases, 2015, https://www.youtube.com/watch?v=iI5Bhf-mZp8&feature=youtube_gdata_player.

[2] Barnard and Associates, *A Low-Fat Vegan Diet Improves Glycemic Control and Cardiovascular Risk Factors in a Randomized Clinical Trial in Individuals with Type 2 Diabetes.*, Diabetes Care, Volume 29, August 2006, http://www.nealbarnard.org/pdfs/Diabetes-Care.pdf.

[3] Neal D Barnard et al., "A Low-Fat Vegan Diet and a Conventional Diabetes Diet in the Treatment of Type 2 Diabetes: A Randomized, Controlled, 74-Wk Clinical trial1234," *The American Journal of Clinical Nutrition* 89, no. 5 (May 2009): 1588S – 1596S, doi:10.3945/ajcn.2009.26736H. http://www.ncbi.nlm.nih.gov/pmc/articles/PMC2677007/

Introduction

Diabetes is a difficult illness to diagnose without going to your doctor. So it is best to see your doctor right away if you feel like you are having symptoms of diabetes. Some of these early symptoms include: frequent urination, excessive thirst, tiredness, blurry vision, cuts that don't heal and tingling sensations in your fingers or toes.

If you or a loved one, is experiencing any of these symptoms you should talk with your primary care doctor. They will do some blood work to help determine if your symptoms are early signs of diabetes.

If you are already struggling with diabetes then you know all these symptoms very well. These things might be happening to you on a daily basis, which is making you seek out a way to reverse your diabetes.

First, let's look at some of the symptoms of diabetes. Then, we will discuss some of the important ways a low-fat vegan diet can help eliminate your diabetes forever!

This is a battle you have to be ready to fight. It will take great effort on your part to fight and reverse your diabetes. But if you are willing to put in the effort you will get a huge reward in the end: a healthy life without diabetes.

About Diabetes

Diabetes mellitus (DM), commonly referred to simply as diabetes, is a group of metabolic diseases in which there are high blood sugar levels over a prolonged period.[1]

Diabetes is caused either by the pancreas not producing enough insulin or the cells of the body not responding properly to the insulin produced. There are three main types of diabetes mellitus:

1. Type 1 DM results from the body's failure to produce enough insulin. This form was previously referred to as "insulin-dependent diabetes mellitus" (IDDM) or "juvenile diabetes". The cause is unknown.[2]

2. Type 2 DM begins with insulin resistance, a condition in which cells fail to respond to insulin properly. As the disease progresses, a lack of insulin may also develop.[3] This form was previously referred to as "non insulin-dependent diabetes mellitus" (NIDDM) or "adult-onset diabetes". The primary cause is excessive body weight and not enough exercise.[4]

3. Gestational diabetes is the third main form and occurs when pregnant women without a previous history of diabetes develop a high blood glucose level.[5]

If you are suffering from some of these signs of diabetes now is the time to take control of your life and start fighting against your diabetes. If you have pre-diabetes or early diabetes you can make the changes necessary to see significant results very quickly. If you have had diabetes for a long time, it might take longer to see the results.

Now is the time to start the process of reversing your disease. With this guide you will be able to understand your disease better and get control of your diet to make the great changes necessary to better your health.

Diabetes is a serious illness and you have to take it seriously. As of

---

[1] „About diabetes". World Health Organization. Retrieved 4 April 2014.
[2] „Diabetes Fact sheet N°312". WHO. October 2013. Retrieved 25 March 2014.
[3] RSSDI textbook of diabetes mellitus. (Rev. 2nd ed.). New Delhi: Jaypee Brothers Medical Publishers. 2012. p. 235.
[4] „Diabetes Fact sheet N°312".
[5] „Diabetes Fact sheet N°312". WHO. October 2013. Retrieved 25 March 2014.

2014, an estimated 387 million people have diabetes worldwide,[6] with type 2 diabetes making up about 90% of the cases.[7,8]

People die from diabetes! It can change how your heart functions, blood pressure, circulation, kidneys, liver and many other functions.

People who suffer from diabetes often have many other illnesses that change their ability to function on a daily basis. As diabetes becomes more advanced you may even face huge medical hurdles. Some people with diabetes end up getting their toes, fingers or limbs amputated because of complications from their diabetes.

This is not an illness you need to be messing around with. This is your life and you need to take control of it. Do not let another moment go by without being in control of your diabetes. **Start taking the steps you need to in order to reverse your diabetes now.**

---

[6] „Update 2014". IDF. International Diabetes Federation. Retrieved 29 November 2014.
[7] Williams textbook of endocrinology (12th ed.). Philadelphia: Elsevier/Saunders. pp. 1371–1435. ISBN 978-1-4377-0324-5.
[8] Shi, Yuankai; Hu, Frank B. „The global implications of diabetes and cancer". The Lancet 383 (9933): 1947–8. doi:10.1016/S0140-6736(14)60886-2. PMID 24910221.

Symptoms of high blood sugar

Frequent Trips to the Bathroom

We all have those days where we run off to the bathroom a few more times than normal. But if you notice yourself making frequent trips over several days or several weeks, it may be something to discuss with your doctor. Keep a journal of how much you are drinking and how often you are urinating so you have some information to show your doctor.

Overly Thirsty

If you are overly thirsty and drinking more fluid it is likely you will also be using the bathroom more often. There are other reasons your body might be thirsty, not just as an early sign of diabetes. Thirst can indicate dehydration or even a normal reaction to certain medications. If you feel like you are excessively thirsty and it is something new, it may be an early sign of diabetes though; so go see your doctor.

Tiredness

As adults, and certainly as parents, we get tired sometimes. It's even possible for us to get a full night sleep and still feel exhausted the next day. The toll of day-to-day life can sometimes increase the need for sleep that your body has. But if you notice yourself becoming tired in the middle of the day, or even after having several days of good sleep, this is something to pay attention to.

Blurry Vision

Sudden blurry vision is a very serious condition and you should go to a doctor or emergency room. But slowly increasing blurred vision that comes and goes away may be an early symptom of diabetes.

This is an often-ignored symptom of other illnesses as well, so just get to the doctor so they can check you out and see what is causing the blurry vision. You need to talk with your doctor right away if you are having this symptom from your diabetes, it is a very serious condition which needs a doctor to look at it to ensure you are healthy.

Wounds that are Not Healing

When your body is busy trying to balance the insulin and glucose in your cells, it cannot work on healing wounds. Some people will notice this as the first sign of diabetes. A wound can sometimes take a week or two to heal normally, but if you notice your cut is taking more time than that, talk with your doctor. Keep the wound clean and dry and write down how long it has been healing. It might also be a good time to look at the other early symptoms to see if you are having any of those.

Tingling in Extremities

It is normal for your foot to fall asleep if you have been sitting on it or your arm to feel numb when you wake up after sleeping on it. Early signs of diabetes that including tingling in your extremities will not be associated with how you slept or sat on your limb. Instead, you might notice tingling when you are sitting at work or numbness when you are driving.

Early signs of diabetes may not show at all, these are just some typical symptoms. If you feel like you have any of these, or if you are just not feeling right and think something might be going on, see your doctor. Many illnesses that have similar symptoms as diabetes are just as important to catch as early as possible.

1|
Diabetes and Your Body: The Good, Bad, and Evil

Fighting diabetes involves lifestyle and diet changes. If you are able to take these steps before you get full blown diabetes you can prevent the progression of the disease. The top five steps to take include: exercise, drinking water, reducing sugary foods, regular doctor visits and eating more vegetables.

If you are able to incorporate these steps into your lifestyle and diet you will be making the necessary changes to help avoid developing diabetes. Talk with your doctor right away to get your baseline and see if they agree with the steps needed to prevent diabetes.

Diabetes will slowly progress through your body and take a serious toll on how your organs function. Your liver, kidneys, eyes and brain will all function poorly as your diabetes progresses.

Some of the things you need to be aware of and start changing right away include:

The Importance of a Vegan Diet

Vegetarian and vegan diets offer significant benefits for diabetes management. In observational studies, individuals following vegetarian diets are about half as likely to develop diabetes, compared with non-vegetarians. In clinical trials in individuals with type 2 diabetes, low-fat vegan diets improve glycemic control to a greater extent than conventional diabetes diets. Although this effect is primarily attributable to greater weight loss, evidence also suggests that reduced intake of saturated fats and high-glycemic-index foods, increased intake of dietary fiber and vegetable protein, reduced intramyocellular lipid concentrations, and decreased iron stores mediate the influence of plant-based diets on glycemia. Vegetarian and vegan diets also improve plasma lipid concentrations and have been shown to reverse atherosclerosis progression. In clinical studies, the reported acceptability of vegetarian and vegan diets is comparable to other therapeutic regimens. The presently available literature indicates that vegetarian and vegan diets present potential advantages for the management of type 2 diabetes.[9]

Lowering Your Fat Intake

A low-fat vegan diet improves glycemic control and cardiovascular risk factors in a randomized clinical trial in individuals with type 2 diabetes.

Objective of the research: Investigate whether a low-fat vegan diet improves glycemic control and cardiovascular risk factors in individuals with type 2 diabetes. *Conclusion of the research:* Both a low-fat vegan diet and a diet based on ADA guidelines improved glycemic and lipid control in type 2 diabetic patients. **These improvements were greater with a low-fat vegan diet.**[10]

Train yourself to think low-fat when you eat, shop and order in restaurants.

Reducing Refined Sugar Foods

The amount of sugar your body is taking in on a daily basis can significantly affect the way your body reacts to sugar in the long run. If you are pre-diabetic it is essential that you reduce your sugar intake as

---

[9] Vegetarian and vegan diets in type 2 diabetes management. Nutr Rev. 2009 May;67(5):255-63. doi: 10.1111/j.1753-4887.2009.00198.x. Barnard ND1, Katcher HI, Jenkins DJ, Cohen J, Turner-McGrievy G.
http://www.ncbi.nlm.nih.gov/pubmed/19386029
[10] Diabetes Care. 2006 Aug;29(8):1777-83. Barnard ND1, Cohen J, Jenkins DJ, Turner-McGrievy G, Gloede L, Jaster B, Seidl K, Green AA, Talpers S.
http://www.ncbi.nlm.nih.gov/pubmed/16873779

soon as possible.

The most important foods to avoid are candy and other sugary snacks. These hold very little nutritional value and can easily be removed from your diet. Other foods that quickly turn into sugars are white carbohydrates, which include foods like potatoes and rice. These foods are appropriate in small amounts but in large amounts they overwhelm your system and quickly turn into sugars in your body.

Starches and Vegetables

Eating more starches (potatoes, beans, corn) and vegetables is the perfect way to decrease your appetite and increase the nutrients in your diet. Incorporate starches and vegetables into your daily meals as much as possible and it will reduce hunger and help your body feel great. Both raw and cooked vegetables are great choices for your diet and will help you fill up so you are not eating as much sugar and other foods.

Getting rid of all the negative foods which are contributing to your diabetes is easier said than done. Your body has come to depend on these unhealthy foods and will start to withdraw as you take these foods away. It is essential that you are building up your vitamins and minerals with as many healthy vegetables as you can during the process of stopping your unhealthy foods. Keep thinking about how great you are going to feel when you have reversed your diabetes!

As you cut out sugar from your diet in the form of refined carbohydrates, refined sugars and processed foods, your body will feel energetic. Still, it is important to give yourself plenty of extra time to rest and for sleeping. Sleep is a necessary part to your body giving up on the unhealthy foods and you starting to eat more healthy foods.

Think about how all your friends and family will be coming to you for help. How they will look up to you for all the hard work you have done. This is your chance to show everyone you are ready to make a change.

Exercise

When you exercise it forces your body to use up insulin at a higher rate. To help prevent Type 2 diabetes, you should incorporate a healthy exercise routine into your daily lifestyle. While it is not necessary to exercise every single day, it is helpful to exercise at least three times per week.

Your body will stimulate the liver to produce the correct amount of insulin to help burn off sugars. Exercise can also be an important tool to incorporate after eating large meals. When you eat a large meal your body may struggle to produce the correct amount of insulin, by walking right after your meal your body will be stimulated to produce the insulin.

Water, not Other Drinks

Switching out soda for water is an essential step in stopping diabetes before it starts. Sugary sodas are a well know culprit for diabetes, but diet soda can also contribute to your body not operating as well as it should. Do not let your thirst for sugary drinks overcome your knowledge of how bad these types of drinks are for your body. Your body does not need these drinks and they are actually making your diabetes worse much faster than any of the foods you are eating.

Switch out all your soda drinks for water to give your body the necessary hydration it needs to flush out toxins and operate at its peak. Water also helps your metabolism function and will increase the rate at which your body is able to process food. Water is essential in your fight against diabetes.

Regular Doctors Visits

Visiting with your primary care doctor on a regular basis can help keep you from continuing down the path to Type 2 diabetes. Your doctor can help you see the early warning signs of diabetes so you can make changes quickly to prevent full-blown diabetes from setting in.

Talk with your doctor regularly about your concerns and any changes to your diet or eating regimen that you plan to make. It may be helpful to get a baseline A1C blood test drawn so you can compare them yearly and keep track of your progress. Your doctor is your greatest ally in the fight against diabetes, be sure to talk with them on a regular basis about your concerns and questions.

You need your doctor to be able to guide you in this fight to reverse your diabetes. So find a doctor you like and who is supportive of your efforts to get off of medications.

2 | Why High Fat Diets Cause Diabetes

Type 2 diabetes occurs when the body does not produce a sufficient amount of insulin or is unable to use insulin in the proper manner. It is an unsubstantiated myth that the cause of diabetes is attributed to sugar consumption. Diabetes, more specifically type 2 diabetes, is not caused by eating too much sugar, but is instead triggered by genetics and lifestyle influences. This typically happens to those that are overweight, obese, above 40 years of age, or already at risk due to a family history of the ailment. In recent years, research studies have shifted gears and begun to focus on high fat diets as a cause of diabetes and examined how specific dietary changes can reverse the disorder.

Diabetes and insulin resistance are metabolic disorders. Research and experiments have revealed that this particular group of diseases is growing and indicated that they are linked to low-grade inflammation. Studies, conducted in both human and mice subjects, have confirmed that a diet high in fat will generate inflammation. The inflammation will promote diabetes, or other metabolic diseases, and generate circulating levels of lipopolysaccharide (LPS), a plasma endotoxin. LPS originates in the digestive system. Analyses have shown that meals where 33% or more of the calories come from fat will increase LPS levels and subsequently create metabolic issues.

Professional groups, such as the American Heart Association, American Diabetes Association, and the United States Department of Agriculture advocate that individuals derive no more than 30% of their calories from fat sources. In addition to diabetes, consuming too much fat, especially saturated fats and cholesterol, will increase the risk of numerous other diseases and disorders such as increased blood cholesterol, heart disease, and various cancers. Diets high in fat will also eventually lead to weight gain and possible obesity. Most patients who are newly diagnosed with Type 2 diabetes are overweight or obese.

Nature Medicine published a study that described a conduit through which high-fat diets are linked to a molecular event sequence and result in the onset of diabetes. In this pathway, increased levels of fat impede two essential transcription factors, or proteins that switch genes on and off. These factors are FoxA2 and HNF1A and are required for the production of GnT-4a glycosyltransferase. GnT-4a's ability to function is severely reduced when FoxA2 and HNF1A are not performing their role properly. These researchers fed mice a diet high in fat and discovered that the mice's beta cells could not correctly detect or respond to blood glucose. Howard Hughes Medical Institute, in Maryland, has discovered a link between a Western-style diet, which is high in fat, and the inception of diabetes. The researchers conducted studies in mice that revealed a diet high in fat would disrupt the production of insulin and result in the classic markers of Type 2 diabetes. These scientists reported that the high-fat diet suppressed the activity of the enzyme GnT-4a glycosyltransferase in the mice. By inhibiting this single enzyme, insulin production was disrupted and led to Type 2 diabetes.

Recent results from studies conducted by the Finnish Diabetes Prevention Study and the Diabetes Prevention Program also confirm the notion that high-fat diets will impair insulin function or encourage insulin resistance. Their findings delve a bit further and suggest that any dietary factor that promotes weight gain also advances the likelihood of the eventual development of diabetes. These particular studies focused on high intakes of processed meats and saturated fat as links to an increased risk of Type 2 diabetes.

New findings that favor dietary changes as treatment for Type 2 diabetes resulted from a detailed study and comparison of diets from cultures around the world. In Japan, for example, the traditional diet is based on foods that come largely from plant sources. Studies revealed that in Japan, and other countries where diets are plant-derived, diabetes is rare. In the United States, and other countries with Western-style diets, meals are fattier and meatier and cause the body to be more insulin resistant. Interventions that include dietary alterations and the addition of physical activity can lead to weightloss and the eventual prevention, postponement, or reversal of diabetes.

Clinical studies have demonstrated that a low-fat, plant-based diet will improve insulin resistance, aid in weight loss, and reduce blood sugar, blood pressure, and cholesterol. Diets derived from plants are, by design, very low in saturated fat. This simple diet change could reverse diabetes without portion control or exhausting exercises. The basic prescription is to simply avoid all animal products (fats and proteins) and eliminate vegetable oils.

Dr. Neal Barnard, the founder and president of the Physician's Committee for Responsible Medicine and professor of medicine at George Washington University School of Medicine in Washington, D.C., has extensively studied the concept of dietary interventions as a treatment for Type 2 diabetes. Dr. Barnard suggests attempting diet changes first before prescribing any medications for the treatment of diabetes. In one of Barnard's studies, teams from George Washington University, the University of Toronto, and the University of North Carolina teamed up together. Their research focused on the effect a vegan diet had on weight loss and diabetes when compared to the standard American diet. For 22 weeks, participants were divided into two groups and asked to consume a specific diet. One group followed a plant-based, vegan diet and the others dined on a Western-style diet with certain modifications and recommendations. At the conclusion of the study, the vegan group's participants had lost an average of 14 pounds each and 43% were able to stop or lower dosages of medications prescribed to control their diabetes. Those that were following a modified standard American diet lost an average of 6.8 pounds. Only 26% of participants in the second group were able to stop or reduce their prescription medications. Barnard's conclusion is that the vegan diet actually reworks what goes on within an individual's cells and will eventually repair the body and reverse diabetes. Based on this particular study and others, in 2007, Barnard published a book expounding on his findings. *Dr. Neal Barnard's Program for Reversing Diabetes*[4] details how diabetes responds radically to a diet low in fat and void of animal products and explains that this change will reestablish how the body uses insulin.[11]

---

[11]

http://humanfoodproject.com/can-a-high-fat-paleo-diet-cause-obesity-and-diabetes/, Can a high fat Paleo Diet cause obesity and diabetes?, Human Food Project

http://care.diabetesjournals.org/content/25/3/620.full, Dietary Fat and the Development of Type 2 Diabetes, American Diabetes Association

"Type 2 diabetes is not a disease. Type 2 diabetes is an adaptation. It's a survival adaptation that the body takes."[5]
~ John McDougall, M.D.

Dr. John McDougall shares how he treats and helps his patients revert diabetes with diet:

Part 1 www.youtube.com/watch?v=6u4IiVbPdKk

Part 2 www.youtube.com/watch?v=WGPO5Fg8_4s

---

[4] Neal Barnard, MD, "Dr. Neal Barnard's Program for Reversing Diabetes," n.d., http://www.pcrm.org/shop/byNealBarnard/dr-barnards-program-for-reversing-diabetes.

[5] *HIGHLIGHTS: Dr. McDougall's Dietary Therapy: An Online Course for Reversing Common Diseases*, 2015, https://www.youtube.com/watch?v=iI5Bhf-mZp8&feature=youtube_gdata_player.

---

http://www.eurekalert.org/pub_releases/2005-12/hhmi-rdh122105.php, Researchers discover how a high-fat diet causes type 2 diabetes, EurekAlert

http://beaker.sanfordburnham.org/2011/08/how-fatty-diets-cause-diabetes/, How fat and obesity cause diabetes, Sanford Burnham Medical Research Institute

http://www.joslin.org/info/4_Myths_About_Diabetes.html, Four Myths about Diabetes, Joslin Diabetes Center

http://pcrm.org/health/diabetes-resources/the-vegan-diet-how-to-guide-for-diabetes, The Vegan Diet How-To Guide for Diabetes, Physicians Committee for Responsible Medicine

http://www.huffingtonpost.com/neal-barnard-md/a-prescription-for-a-plan_b_6178622.html, A Prescription for a Plant-Based Diet Can Help Reverse Diabetes, Huffington Post

http://www.nealbarnard.org/, Dr. Neal Barnard's Website

http://abcnews.go.com/Health/Diabetes/wireStory?id=2244647, Vegan diet reverses diabetes symptoms, study finds, ABC News

http://www.pennmedicine.org/health_info/nutrition/fat.html, Fat in Your Diet, Penn Medicine

3|
Basics

Trying to get healthier and become a vegetarian may seem like a good idea until you start trying to figure out all the basics of what you can and cannot eat. The basics of being a vegetarian are that you are giving up eating meat products and all other food products that are from animals.

Instead of eating animal products your diet concentrates on starchy low-fat plant-based foods. Once you start down the path of vegetarianism you will quickly get the hang of all the do's and don'ts associated with this eating lifestyle.

Changing to a vegan diet is better for your health than just reversing diabetes. This type of diet will help reduce many ailments in your body. You will want to keep up with this diet even after you have reversed your diabetes. Plant-based diets can reduce or eliminate diabetes according to the U.S. Department of Health and Human Services.[12]

By eating a diet full of vegetables, legumes, and other nutritious plant foods, you'll be getting a full range of nutrients without any of the harmful additives or fats that are often a part of the average meat eater's diet. Most people tend to neglect plant foods even though these are essential sources of vitamins and minerals that you simply can't find in meat. Migraine or headache sufferers who go on vegan diets frequently discover relief from their migraines. Reduction in dairy, meat, and eggs is often tied to alleviation of allergy symptoms. Many vegans report much

---

[12] http://newsinhealth.nih.gov/issue/Jul2012/Feature1

fewer runny noses and congestion problems. Eating a healthy vegan diet has also shown to prevent a number of diseases (cardiovascular disease, high cholesterol, high blood pressure, diabetes, macular degeneration, fungus, cataracts, acid reflux disease, arthritis, osteoporosis, eczema, chronic fatigue syndrome, asthma). Your weight will go down, your skin will turn into beautiful, clear, healthy-looking skin (some people call it "Glow"), your whole body will be working more efficiently, and you'll just feel better overall.

Meat

As a vegan, you will have to give up all meat. This means no hamburgers, steaks, chicken sandwiches or any other meat. Giving up eating meat is a hard thing to do if you are typically using this as your main protein source. You can start with giving up meat at your morning meals, then lunch and finally dinner. Do this slowly over a few weeks to give yourself time to adjust to the changes.

Animal Products

There are a wide variety of other animal products that we are constantly consuming in our daily life. Milk and eggs are just a couple of these animal products. Becoming a vegan means you are going to be giving up these products, as well as meat. There are vegan and vegetarian options you can find for these food products if you shop at your local health food store. Pick the low-fat versions.

Eat Plenty of Starches!

Getting enough starch is an essential part of staying healthy while on your vegan diet. Starchy foods should be 90% of your daily intake and thus be included in every single meal and snack you are eating if you want to stay healthy and reverse diabetes without drugs. It is important, however, to make sure to eat the correct kinds of starches. Eating the wrong types of starches would have the opposite effect of what we are looking for.

- **Grains**

Whole grains are the best source of grains to include in your vegetarian diet. Although you can get grains from a wide variety of sources that include white carbohydrates, it is best to try and consume only whole grains.

You can eat brown rice, pasta, noodles, and oats all made of pure whole grains. These whole grains will provide your body the carbohydrates it needs to function at its best while also offering a higher content of nutrients from the whole grains.

- **Legumes**

This is a great source of protein if you are a vegetarian. Legumes include foods like peas, soybeans, chickpeas and beans. You can eat these raw or get them from a can. You can add legumes to your salads and almost any other recipe to increase the amount of protein you are getting in your diet. Eating plenty of legumes will help you maintain a diet that is rich in protein and legumes also have high iron content.

Eating a vegetarian diet is not as hard as you might think but it will take some time to get used to it. There are plenty of unhealthy foods that vegetarians eat as well as the healthy foods listed here. Try to keep this healthy food list as much as possible to ensure you are exposing yourself to the healthiest foods for your body.

Vegetables and Fruits

One of the best sources of food for the vegetarian lifestyle is to eat plenty of vegetables and fruits throughout your day. Vegetables are a great source of protein, vitamins, and minerals. Eating dark leafy vegetables will give you the highest concentration of nutrients. **Limit the amount of fruits you are eating to 2 to 3 servings a day as they contain a high amount of natural sugars.**

There is a lot of research available that discuss how important it is to eat **salads and fruits** on a daily basis. Eating salads can help lower your blood sugar because you are filling your body with healthy lettuce to keep your body busy processing your foods.

Eating fruit is an important part of eating a healthy diet, but you should be aware of how much and how often you can eat fruit due to its effects on your blood sugar. Check out this video on *How to Eat Fruit for Diabetics:* www.youtube.com/watch?v=7PT2vdnwwV0. It talks about the importance to adding salad/fiber to the fruit diet to reduce blood sugar levels.

Another great resource for you in helping you understand the importance of fruits is *Overcame Type 2 Diabetes in 2 Weeks on a High Fruit Raw Diet:* www.youtube.com/watch?v=o9fXi2YOEw4

How Often to Eat

You will notice a need to eat more often, especially when you first start with your vegan diet. Healthy foods like fruits, vegetables, and whole grains do not take as long to process through your body, so you will become hungry quicker than you would if you were eating animal meats.

To fight off this hunger it is helpful to make up some snacks and keep them with you throughout your day. Simple protein-based snacks like nuts are a great way to have a quick bite to eat and curb your hunger feelings. You can also cut up vegetables and fruits and keep them in containers for easy on-the-go options.

Dining Out

It used to be incredibly hard to be a vegan and go to a normal restaurant. But not anymore, in today's world it is easier than ever to eat a vegan diet and visit traditional dining out locations. You will notice many healthy options on the menu and plenty of choices for you that are vegan friendly.

If you do not see specific menu items that are vegan you can easily turn a salad from any menu into a vegan option by asking for them to leave off the animal meat and cheese from the salad. A simple green salad with vegetables will act as your go-to meal when you are traveling and dining out.

Make sure and talk with your friends and family so they can help you stick to your vegan diet and perhaps even ask them to try out a vegan or vegetarian restaurant with you.

Protein

Protein is not only found in animals. Many plant foods are loaded with protein and it's actually extremely easy to get your full daily requirement of protein without eating a single animal product. Grains, legumes, beans, nuts, and seeds are all tiny protein powerhouses. **It's just as easy to get enough protein with a vegan diet as it is with**

any other diet.

In this guide we will include some of the most popular vegan fresh foods and the amount of protein they contain. You should use this guide to help you plan your snacks and meals to ensure you are getting the recommended daily amount of protein in your diet.

Women and men typically need between 40 and 50 grams of protein on a daily basis. Some recources claim even less. Your recommended daily amount of protein is based on your weight and you can discuss this with your doctor to get the most accurate number for you at your current weight.

4|
Cutting Out the Evil

If one or more members of your family have diabetes it is important to know how to manage diabetes as a family and not just individually. Making your kitchen a safe place for family members with diabetes is an important aspect to maintaining healthy blood glucose levels.

Educating the whole family about diabetes symptoms and issues is also extremely important; this can include signs of low blood sugar, daily eating habits, and parameters for when to ask for help. Working together as a family can make diabetes a much more manageable medical condition.

Making the necessary changes to your diet to reverse your diabetes will take the help of your whole family. You will need their support so let them help you with every step of this process.

The more poor food choices you are cutting out, the more room you will have for the good food choices that you want to start adding to your diet. Building your good food choices will take time and so will getting rid of your bad food choices.

Diabetes Friendly Kitchen

Whether you have a toddler, teen or adult in the house with diabetes, a kitchen filled with safe foods is essential for managing diabetes. Eating the right combination of fats, proteins and carbohydrates is such an important aspect of a healthy diabetic diet. Families can make their kitchen diabetes friendly by keeping lots of healthy fruits and vegetables around. Take the time to cut up veggies and put in small containers in the fridge and this will make them more appealing to kids on the go.

Keep the sugary junk food out of the kitchen. No one really needs to have a Twinkie or donut, whether you have diabetes or not. Just don't even purchase this kind of junk food for your kitchen, it is extremely appealing to someone suffering from diabetes and it is extremely unsafe for them also. Instead of junk food like that, make healthy pumpkin bars or trail mix and keep it in snack-size baggies that are pre-portioned out.

Symptoms of Low Blood Sugar and What to Do

Low blood sugar or hypoglycemia is a dangerous side effect of having too much glucose in the body. Any family member who uses glucose on a daily basis is at risk for having an insulin reaction that results in hypoglycemia. This is very dangerous and as a family every member should be aware of the warning signs and the best way to treat low blood sugar. As you change your eating habits it is essential that you monitor your blood sugar levels on a frequent basis.

Symptoms of low blood sugar include sweating, shakiness, fast heartbeat, dizziness, and sleepiness. It is important to keep small amounts of simple carbohydrates available that can be used during a hypoglycemic incident. Miniature regular sodas, orange juice in small child size containers, honey and glucose tablets are all commonly used to bring glucose levels up during a hypoglycemic incident. Your family needs to be aware of these symptoms so they can help.

Eating Habits

Small regular meals are an important aspect of managing diabetes. This might mean avoiding large dinners, which can be difficult for families to understand unless they work together to plan meals that are more diabetic friendly. Instead of eating a large dinner plan to have a salad earlier in the evening, and protein with vegetables a few hours later. This way you still get all the meal, but it is spread out over a period of time to help manage blood sugar spikes.

Asking for Help

As a family, it is important to work together in preparing your home and lifestyle to manage diabetes. Remember to ask your family for help if there is a particular area you are struggling with. If you need more help in the morning planning a healthy breakfast, or during the day while at work, take the time to work as a family and help each other make life as good as it can be.

Living with diabetes takes some energy and adjustments. But if you work together you can manage diabetes as a family. Make meal planning and preparation fun and work to find foods that are healthy and diabetic friendly. If you still need more support, check out your local hospital or health center, many have diabetes groups where you can meet other families going through the same issues and concerns as you are.

Grocery Shopping

When you first start eating a vegan low-fat diet you will notice there are areas of your grocery store that you just cannot go into anymore. The entire middle section!

This will be difficult at first, but you will soon find your comfort areas where all the good food is. You will spend most of your time in the produce section. Find a store that you are comfortable with their produce quality so you can get all your fruits and vegetables from one place.

Another area of the store where you will frequent is the health food area. Many stores are starting to have a specific area that is designated to healthier foods. This area may include whole grain foods, organic products and other foods that you should be checking out.

Friends and Family

This might seem like an area that you wouldn't dare get rid of people out of, but it may be necessary to distance yourself from some of the people in your life.

As you start eating a vegan low-fat diet, there are going to be people in your life that do not support this change. Some of your friends and family may not be ready to make the same changes in their life so they will have a difficult time supporting your changes.

These friends and family will make it harder for you to stick to your goal of reversing your diabetes because they may start to sabotage your progress. This is not intentionally done, but sometimes, unintentionally, people we love will sabotage our progress.

If you start to notice any friends or family members that are not supportive of you, it is time to distance yourself from them. You need a clear head during this reversal process and you only want people around that are going to encourage and support you.

Reversing diabetes is hard enough; you need to keep people around you that can help! Supportive and caring people around you are exactly what you need to make it through this process.

5 | Building up Your Army of Superfoods

If you have been struggling to get your diabetes under control you probably have been visiting with your doctor pretty regularly. Your doctor has probably made suggestions on healthy eating habits that can help you get your diabetes under control.

The more starchy foods you can include in your diet the better it will be. Starch is the cornerstone to eating as a vegan and should be included in as many of your meals as possible.

As you change your eating to help you reverse your diabetes, make sure to take small steps so you are not feeling overwhelmed by the food changes. Small changes will most likely last longer than if you were trying to change all of your eating habits all at once.

Transitioning your diet to a vegan food plan is an excellent way to increase your ability to keep your diabetes stable. Following a vegan food diet gives you more vitamins, leaves less room for junk food, causes a reduction in your weight, and helps to lower blood sugars. You do not have to convert to a total vegan food diet all at once, but making small raw food changes can result in a big change to your diabetes health.

Many people with diabetes suffer from high blood pressure also. As you start to build up your good foods it is helpful to add foods that will help your diabetes as well as your blood pressure.

The U.S. National Institute of Health reports did a study showing the control over diabetes when a low-fat vegan diet was used.[13]

Adding green vegetables to your starch based diet is a necessity, these foods are high in potassium which naturally helps to lower your blood pressure and keep your blood sugar levels under control.

Green vegetables are also low in calories and sodium so they are the perfect food for your overall health as well as your heart health. Taking the time to change your diet and incorporate more green vegetables can show significant results in lowering your blood pressure, lowering blood sugars and increasing your body's ability to fight diabetes.

Adding these super foods and the ones listed in later chapters will ensure your body is operating at its peak. Keep these in mind when you are making salads to really boost the nutritional value of your salad.

Many of the influential people in the world of diabetes and health are all saying the same thing about what you should be eating. John Mackey, Co-Founder, Co-CEO of Whole Foods Market, said: "The one [program] that's had the biggest impact in terms of really changing people's lives [...]: we work with 4 different doctors around the country and their programs are all 99% alike. They are whole food plant based diets that significantly reduce any kind of refined sugars, that don't have oil in them, that virtually have no animal food and are all plant based. The four programs, each of them, is miraculous. The results are significant in just seven days. [...] The human body is more resilient, I had no idea. It can heal itself fairly rapidly if we just stop poisoning it. It wants to heal. Only we just keep insulting it with poison day after day after day. But turn the poison off, give him healthy nutritious food, body starts to heal, starts to return to a healthy state and healthy condition. Disease takes reverse. It's astounding."[14]

---

[13] www.ncbi.nlm.nih.gov/pmc/articles/PMC2677007/
[14] www.youtube.com/watch?v=Vw5JVkGNMUc

The Super Foods

Sweet Potato

A simple way to begin eating healthier is by adding sweet potatoes into you diet in order to replace your "regular" potato intake. Many find sweet potatoes so delicious that they do not have an issue with making them their go-to potato. Now, it's ok to eat a nice good old baked potato once in a while, but when looking at the greater scheme of things, a sweet potato in a better choice when looking for a nutrient-rich super food.

Sweet potatoes can be used as a substitute in just about any recipe that calls for regular potatoes. They are packed with vitamins, minerals, fibers, antioxidents and even have anti-inflamatory properties.

Potato

Potatoes have gotten a pretty bad reputation, but the truth is that they are not entirely bad for you when eaten correctly. French fries, potato chips, baked potatoes soaked in butter and sour cream are all examples of ways you should not be eating potatoes. The truth of the matter is that a baked Russet potato, with no added fats and the skin on, is low in sodium, higher in potassium than a banana, a good source of fiber and has no fat and no cholesterol.

Beans

Beans are not only good for the waistline, but they are great for disease prevention as well. Today, they are seen as more than just a substitute for meat. The latest dietary guidelines recommend that we triple our current intake of beans from only 1 cup per week to 3 cups per week. So what makes them so good for us? They are high in fiber and water content. This means that they help you feel fuller faster, and in turn help you to cut out unnecessary calories without feeling deprived.

Corn

Other than its delicious sweet flavor, there are many other reason why you should be eating corn. Corn is high in fiber, low in fat and it's a great source of essential nutrients that offer great health benefits. Corn is also high in dietary fiber and helps with digestion. Surprisinglt, corn is a great source of iron and helps to prevent anemia. The list of the benefits you will get from adding corn to your diet is extensive.

Rice

Rice is another food that has gotten a bad reputation, but in reality is very good for you. It is important to remember, however, that when choosing rice, it is better to reach for brown rice than white rice. There are many benefits that brown rice provides: it produces energy, helps to reduce weight, it is rich in fiber, it helps to lower cholesterol, protects against heart disease and much more.

Kale

This dark leafy green vegetable is high in potassium and has very few calories. Instead of eating your salads with regular lettuce, consider switching to kale or a combination of kale and spinach. You can make other things with your kale besides salads. You can drizzle olive oil (sparingly!) and roast your kale to make kale chips in your oven.

Another option is to put kale in a smoothie; you can sneak it into a smoothie of any flavor if you are only adding a small bit. If adding kale to a smoothie or juicing it, remember that kale has a very strong flavor so add a small amount first and progressively increase it to adjust to the flavor.

Kale is a great super food that will be an essential part in your fight to reversing your diabetes. Including kale in as many of your meals as possible will help you feel better and control your blood sugar levels.

Beet Greens

Not your typical salad greens but certainly well worth the purchase if you are trying to increase your potassium levels. Make sure to cut up the entire leaf, including the stem to get the highest amounts of vitamins. Beet greens can also be used in smoothies and juicing, but are best suited for salads.

The stem of the beet greens has a bit of a tart taste, which does not work well with very many smoothie recipes. If you include just one cup of beet greens in your salad you will be adding approximately 290 milligrams of potassium.

Lamb's Quarters Plant

This unique plant is delicious when steamed and added to salads. It is almost twice as rich in potassium as beet greens and easy to add a great deal of potassium to any meal. You can also add Lamb's quarters to your salads and blend it in with other vegetables that are rich in potassium. This contains approximately 500 milligrams of potassium per cup.

Bok Choy

If you like to eat Chinese food then you already know how delicious bok choy can be. The dark green part of the bok choy has the most potassium and is where the health benefits lie. One serving of bok choy contains more potassium than a banana, 541 milligrams in one cup. There is a wide variety of bok choy available and it is grown locally throughout the United States and Canada. This dark leafy green vegetable can be added to almost any dish once it is diced up.

Salads

You should be incorporating salads into at least one meal per day. Salads are a great way to mix all your vegetables and get a huge surge of energy from the nutrients. If eating salads, or vegetables is difficult for you, you can try mixing things up a little bit.

Chop up all your salad ingredients very small. This includes kale, broccoli, spinach, cauliflower and any other vegetables you want. Finely chop up one apple and mix it into the salad. This will give you a slight sweet taste and make your vegetables unrecognizable because they are so finely chopped up. In order to lower your blood pressure, you will need to make changes to your diet right away.

It is necessary to cut out as much sodium as possible and to start increasing the amount of potassium you are taking in.

You can increase your potassium by eating more leafy green vegetables such as kale, beet greens, lamb's quarters and bok choy. Try dicing up these vegetables and making a super salad that contains a large amount of potassium. Or if you would prefer to add them to other meals you are making you can add them to casseroles, smoothies, and your morning omelets.

6|
Meal Planning for Low-Fat Super Meals

A vegan diet is full of starchy foods and vegetables. It is essential to make your diet primarily with these items to ensure your body is getting the best low-fat vegan foods. Technically, there are a lot of junk foods that are vegan, you should avoid these and choose foods that are high in protein.

Planning your meals will take time and practice so you can incorporate the healthy low-fat vegan foods while also making meals that you love. Using the list below you can start to become familiar with some of the protein-rich vegan foods that will help you and your family plan your meals.

Research shows that a low-fat vegan diet can help you control your diabetes. So get started today fighting this disease with your meal plans. According to the American Diabetes Association, a low-fat vegan diet improves the body's ability of glycemic control.
(Source: http://www.ncbi.nlm.nih.gov/pmc/articles/PMC2677007/)

Beans (1 Cup Cooked)	Protein (grams)
Lentil	18
Adzuki	17
Cannellini (White Beans)	17
Cranberry Bean	17
Navy Bean	16
Split Peas	16
Anasazi	15
Black Bean	15
Garbanzos (Chick Peas)	15
Kidney Beans	15
Great Northern Beans	15
Lima Beans	15
Pink Beans	15
Black Eyed Peas	14
Mung Beans	14
Pinto Beans	14
Green Peas	9

Grains (1 Cup Cooked)	Protein (grams)
Triticale	25
Millet	8.4
Amaranth	7
Oat, Bran	7
Wild Rice	7
Rye Berries	7
Whole Wheat Couscous	6
Bulgar Wheat	6
Buckwheat	6
Teff	6
Oat Groats	6
Barley	5
Quinoa	5
Brown Rice	5
Spelt	5

Vegetables (1 Cup or as noted)	Protein (grams)
Corn (1 cob)	5
Potato (w/skin)	5
Mushrooms	5
Collard Greens	4
Peas (1/2 cup)	4
Artichoke	4
Avocado	4
Broccoli	4
Brussel Sprouts	4
Fennel	3
Kale	2.5
Asparagus (5 spears)	2
String Beans	2
Beets	2
Sweet Potato	3
Cabbage	2
Carrot	2
Cauliflower	2
Squash	2
Celery	1
Spinach	1
Bell Peppers	1
Cucumber	1
Egg Plant	1
Lettuce	1
Onion (1/2 cup)	1

Nut/Seeds (1/4 Cup or 4 Tbls)	Protein (grams)
Chia Seed	12
Hemp Seed	10
Flax Seed	8
Sunflower Seed	8
Salba	7.4
Almond	7
Pumpkin Seed	7
Sesame Seed	7
Pistachio	6
Walnut	5
Brazil Nut	5
Hazelnut	5
Pine Nut	4
Cashew	4
Chestnut	1

You should use nuts and seeds very sparingly as they're high in total fat. Avoid nuts as a snack. They are natural and contain a lot of protein, but for the most part they are also very high in fat. The one exception is chestnuts, which have only about 8 percent fat.

7|
Doctor Visits & Reversing Diabetes

It is essential that you are taking the time to visit with your doctor regarding your diabetes. Your doctor is an essential part of you being able to reverse your diabetes and take back control of your life. Discuss your vegan eating plans with your doctor and get some preliminary blood work done so you can see what your progress is throughout your new diet plan.

Your doctor may have some concerns about you changing your eating plan, but being open to them and discussing what your process is going to be will be useful. Having a doctor that is on your side will help you feel more comfortable throughout the process. Not all doctors are going to force medications on you. It is possible to find a doctor that will let you start a new diet routine and exercise routine and give you some feedback as to wheter or not they are working.

Depending on how severe your diabetes is, your doctor may suggest that you continue taking your insulin or other medications even after you have made diet changes. It is important to listen to your doctor and follow their recommendations. If you are open with them about your goal to reverse diabetes and get off of medications they will help you reach that goal.

Keeping your food journal and bringing it into your doctors visits will help your doctor understand your new vegan eating plan and how healthy you are eating now.

Dr. George Guthrie, who is certified in Diabetes Education, was one of the first people to talk about drug-free therapy. He talked about diabetic and overweight people suffering from high blood sugar and choosing to change their diets instead of taking medications. After a year of the diet changes rather than using medicine, he saw his first patient become symptom free and no longer diabetic.[15]

Discuss with your doctor if there are any concerns they have about your health or the new diet plan you are starting. Your doctor may ask you to check your blood sugars more often or make some other recommendations to include in your diet.

Reversing diabetes is a long process and you will want to enlist the help of as many people as you can. Your friends and loved ones will, of course, be very supportive, but your doctor is another level of support that can help you continue to understand your illness.

Understanding your diabetes is an essential part to combating it and reversing it. You have to understand what your blood sugar levels are typically at so you know when they are getting better. You have to understand how diabetes has affected your heart, kidneys and liver so you can be aware when those symptoms are getting better.

Your health is nothing to take lightly so it is important you coordinate your care with your doctor and follow all their advice about what you are doing to change your diet and reverse your diabetes.

In order to know if you are reversing your diabetes you will need to be in touch with your doctor on a regular basis. Your doctor will be the person who is able to finally tell you if you have been successfully able to reverse your diabetes.

If you do not have a doctor who is supportive of your fight to get off of diabetes medications it may be necessary to change doctors. You need someone who is ready to reverse diabetes with you! You need a doctor who understands your goals and is ready to support you in reaching your goals, so find one who you can trust in this fight against diabetes.

---

[15] Source: www.youtube.com/watch?v=rVK5fLtPQKI

8|
Fitness and Your Superhero Sidekick

Reversing diabetes takes more than just changing your diet and monitoring your blood sugars. You need to get your body moving and kick your metabolism back into gear. Working out and getting cardiovascular exercise is going to be your superhero sidekick in your fight against diabetes!

When you get a good workout in, your body increases your metabolism and functions better at processing sugars. If you are able to get a daily workout in, your body will continue to increase its ability to fight against diabetes.

Workouts do not need to be long hours at the gym or using crazy fitness equipment. You can get your workout in simply by going for a walk daily or other fun daily activities. Your body needs to move as much as possible during this fight to reverse diabetes.

Walking or Taking Walks

One great way to get started working out is to start walking. If you are new to working out you might want to start by just walking around your block. This might only take a few minutes, but it will get your heart rate up and give you a good starting point. Getting a workout in and your heart rate up will help you in the fight to reverse your diabetes.

As you get more comfortable walking, you can go around your block more than one time. You do not need to do all your exercise at one time. Instead, try walking around your block a couple times throughout your day. Spreading your workout throughout the day will make it easier to complete and it will also give your metabolism a boost at different times in the day.

Keep a log of the total number of minutes you are spending walking, you will soon realize how easy it is to get up to 30 minutes a day of walking. If you feel comfortable, and your doctor agrees, you can continue to increase your walking time up to 60 minutes a day.

There are a wide variety of other exercises that you might also enjoy and will help you burn fat and get your metabolism moving. You will want to pick exercises that are easy on your joints and fun to do.

Swimming is a fun exercise that incorporates your whole body. If you have extra weight to lose, swimming is the perfect exercise because it is a non-impact exercise and will let your joints work hard without damaging them.

In the pool, you can also enjoy just walking up and down the lanes or trying a water aerobics class to keep your interest and give you some variety in your workouts.

Other great ways to workout and enjoy time with your family include going on walks together, bike riding and just playing fun games. You will be amazed at how many calories you burn by simply running around after your children in a game of tag!

Working out does not have to be overwhelming and can be a fun way to spend time with the people you love. Make exercise a part of your daily plan to reverse your diabetes and you will be astonished at how much better you feel throughout the process.

Be sure to take things slow when you first get started and build up to a daily exercise schedule that you feel comfortable with. Your body will give you warning signs when you are tired, listen to those. You are not in a hurry to exercise more than other people, just go at your own pace so you feel comfortable.

Exercising will soon become something you like to do because you will feel better every time you are doing it. As you reverse your diabetes, exercising will get easier and easier. Get moving today so you can fight your diabetes and reverse it.

9 |
Water – the King of all Superheroes

You might not think of water as a huge support when you are fighting diabetes, but it is the King. Drinking enough water is an essential part of your body being able to operate efficiently.

If your body is dehydrated it cannot fully function, so instead it works on the easiest functions first. When you are dehydrated your body will also send a signal to you that often makes you feel hungry, when you are actually dehydrated. Staying hydrated will help you reduce your urge to eat and help you lose weight and reverse your diabetes.

Increasing Your Water

To start increasing your water intake, you can simply try drinking a glass of water before each of your meals and snacks. It does not need to be a large glass of water, just a normal 8 ounce glass of water will be fine.

By starting this process, you will get used to drinking water several times throughout the day. If you are drinking an 8 ounce glass of water 5 times during the day, you will be getting 40 ounces of water; which is close to the 64 ounces which are recommended. Drinking water is key to reversing diabetes and you should take serious steps to drink more water every day.

Tracking Your Water

If you really want to try and increase the amount of water you are drinking on a daily basis you can start keeping track of your water in your food journal or on your phone. There are several health apps for your smartphone that can help you with this, or simply add it to the items you are keeping track of in your journal.

Other Drinks

It may feel like other drinks are the same as drinking water, but they are not. Even drinks that are high in water content like iced tea will flow through your system differently than plain water does. Try to drink plain water as much as possible throughout the day and only drink other drinks in addition to the 64 ounces of water, which is your goal each day.

If you are able to **keep your body fully hydrated** it will be able to function better and process your food more efficiently. Water is the life source of your body and essential to your body operating at its best. Do not let another moment go by without drinking some water and getting your body functioning at its best.

10 | Blood Sugar Monitoring and Journals

In order to see your progress, you are going to have to keep a journal and monitor your blood sugars on a consistent basis. Journaling is a great way to keep yourself accountable and see the changes you are making on a daily basis. In your journal, you will be able to see what was working well for you and what may not have been working very well.

How to Journal

Journaling is the process of keeping track of your diet, and other important things, so you can see what progress you are making. Journaling should be easy so do not make it too complicated, just keep a small notebook or another item to write down the food items you are eating etc. Your journal will be an invaluable tool for you as you progress through your fight to reverse diabetes.

Keeping a journal that is in your smart phone may be the easiest way to keep your journal. If you are using your phone for all other aspects of your life, journaling in there will be very easy. You will want to seperate your posts by the date, but keep them all in one document.

What to Include

In your fight against diabetes, you will need to keep track of the foods you are eating, water you are drinking, exercise and blood sugars.

Writing them down on a calendar or in a fitness app on your phone will work very well. You want to include the basics of what you are eating so you can see what might be helping you have more energy and maybe what makes you not have any energy.

Your journal has the ability to be anything you need it to be. You can include as much or as little information as you would like. If you feel better keeping detailed notes about everything you eat, including the amount and calories, then you can do that. If you want to keep simple notes that just include the name of the food you ate, you can also do that.

Your journal should be useful to you and in order to be useful to you it will need to include information that you find helpful. Keep as much or as little information as you would like. But make sure it will be useful to you when you look back at the information.

Tracking Progress

You can use your journal or an app on your phone to keep track of your progress. An app will probably do this better than your journal because you can see a physical line to show your weight decreasing.

It is important to set your goal for what reversing diabetes will look like for you. Is your goal to get off of all medications? Then you might want to track the decrease in the amount of insulin you are using. If your goal is to lose weight, you might want to track your weight loss in your journal.

Every part of this journal is special and changable to fit your needs. This journal is supposed to help you through this process. So include all the information that you feel will make your journey easier.

Keeping track of your food can feel very overwhelming at first, but you will get use to it. Since our goal isn't specifically to lose weight you do not need to keep track of calories. Also, most of the foods you will be eating are fruits and vegetables so the calories are very minimal.

Monitor your blood sugars throughout the day and put them in your journal so you can see which foods are helping you lower your blood sugars and which ones might be giving you blood sugar spikes. The longer you are eating a vegan diet, the lower you will see your typical blood sugars throughout the day.

Who to Show

This journal is mainly for you to help give yourself insight into the foods you are eating and how they affect your blood sugar levels. You are the person who will be looking at this journal most often so feel comfortable adding everything you would like to the journal.

You may decide to show your journal to your doctor if you would like their input into how a certain food if affecting you and any ideas your doctor may have for helping you make diet changes.

Revisiting your Old Days

As you progress through your fight to reverse diabetes you should take a moment to revisit some of your first days in the journal. Look back to see how hard things were for you then, and how much easier things are now.

Reversing diabetes is a process that will take time and dedication. Your journal is a great way to look back and see the progress you are making in your fight.

11 | Seeing the Reversal of Diabetes

The process of seeing the reversal of your diabetes might start very rapidly as you incorporate the vegan diet into your eating. As soon as you are able to take the processed foods, sugars, and carbohydrates out of your daily eating you will see a significant decrease in your blood sugar levels.

Your body wants to be able to control its blood sugars on a daily basis. It does not want to have high levels or low levels, so when you start feeding your body the nutrient rich food that it needs you will see a huge difference in how your body reacts to blood sugars.

When you add exercise and water to your daily regimen you will also see how your body enjoys having these things around. Your body will become more efficient and better able to respond to the good sugars, like from fruit that are entering your body.

Don't let your body fool you; it is a smart high-tech machine that is just waiting to be filled with high-powered fuel. When you start eating a low-fat vegan diet you will see just how great your body can be:

- You will first start to see a change in the way you are feeling. As you reverse diabetes you might notice you are able to concentrate better on important tasks. You might notice you are able to read a book and enjoy the relaxation it can bring. Your mind will be more focused and you will be able to enjoy all those tasks that you had been avoiding since the high blood sugars were making it too hard to concentrate.

- Another thing you will start to notice is in your journaling. As you keep track of your daily blood sugar levels you will see them slowly decreasing. If you are taking insulin on a regular basis you will notice the decreasing of the amount of insulin you are using on your sliding scale dosing. If you are taking oral diabetes medication you will also want to visit your doctor regularly and show them your daily blood sugar logged numbers so they can determine if any other medication changes need to be made.

- As you reverse your diabetes you will notice your skin start to look clearer. The typical breakouts on your face or body will occur less frequently than they were before. You will notice your skin feeling and looking more vibrant and feeling like it is smoother than you remember it being. It might also appear that dark spots on your skin are lightening and becoming less visible.

- Your body is going through a lot of changes as you reverse diabetes. One of the most visible changes will be losing weight. Not only are you eating a vegan low-fat diet, but you are drinking more water and exercising more than you were before. These lifestyle changes will help you lose weight on a consistent basis. As you are journaling, you might keep track of your weight once per week to help you see this change.

- The clothes you are used to being tight on you will start getting loose. This is a sign that your body is getting rid of the extra water you were keeping in your cells as well as the weight loss that is occurring because of your diet changes.

- As you begin to lose weight, celebrate the changes by purchasing new clothes that help you feel better about your new changing body.

- Your breath and body will smell better. Surprisingly when we are eating a traditional diet, we do not realize how much our breath and body smells. Eating a diet rich in animal products makes our breath and body smell totally awful. As you start eating a vegan diet you will start to notice a fresher smell to your breath and body. Pretty soon you will be able to notice the breath and body of others who are eating meat still and wonder if that is what you smelled like before.

- It is possible you will notice your hair feeling thicker and growing longer than you have seen it before. When you are filling your body with high-powered fruits and vegetables daily, your body is better able to allow for the care and growth of your hair. Longer hair requires it to be healthier, so as your hair becomes healthier you will start to notice it is growing longer and faster than it historically has in the past.

- Nails are a good determining factor for your overall health. Because nail growth is not an essential function, your nails will often grow very minimally when your health is poor. As you become healthier you will notice your nails becoming stronger and growing longer than they have before.

Keeping track of your progress is the most important way you can track the changes going on in your body. Your daily blood sugars will give you the tell-tale signs that your body is starting to reverse your diabetes.

12|

Vegan Recipes

Included in the next chapter, you will get delicious recipes that will help you reverse your diabetes. These recipes are meant to be used to create a healthy 7-day meal plan. Each meal category includes two quick and easy recipes that can be prepared in under 15 minutes. Mix and match according to your lifestyle and create a meal plan that will work for you. Suited for beginners and advanced cooks alike. All recipes come with nutritional information.

Eating a whole-foods diet without animal foods and added oils, less salt and sugar, and very few processed foods dramatically improves the health!

The recipes in this book are based on a purely starch-plant based diet (diet based on whole starches, vegetables, and fruits) without added oils. Cheers to you for bidding goodbye to animal products, to processed foods and to oil!

The recommended low-fat vegan diet is based on scientific research and recommendations by experts such as Dr. Neal Barnard, T. Collin Campbell, Michael McGregor, and Dr. John McDougall.

If you are ready to transform your life and enjoy some delicious vegan recipes, keep reading.

Breakfast

Recipes Included in this Chapter:

1| *Blueberry Pancakes*

2| *French Toast*

3| *Cinnamon Berry Oatmeal*

4| *Spicy Southern Grits*

5| *Blueberry Muffins*

6| *Breakfast Cookies*

7| *Breakfast Tortillas*

1| Blueberry Pancakes

Servings: 6-8 Pancakes

Prep Time: 4 minutes
Cook Time: 10 minutes

    These pancakes are incredibly easy to make (less than fifteen minutes) and are just as incredibly delicious. You can eat them as-is or add some applesauce as a topping. Whip up a batch for some friends and see if they believe that they are vegan.

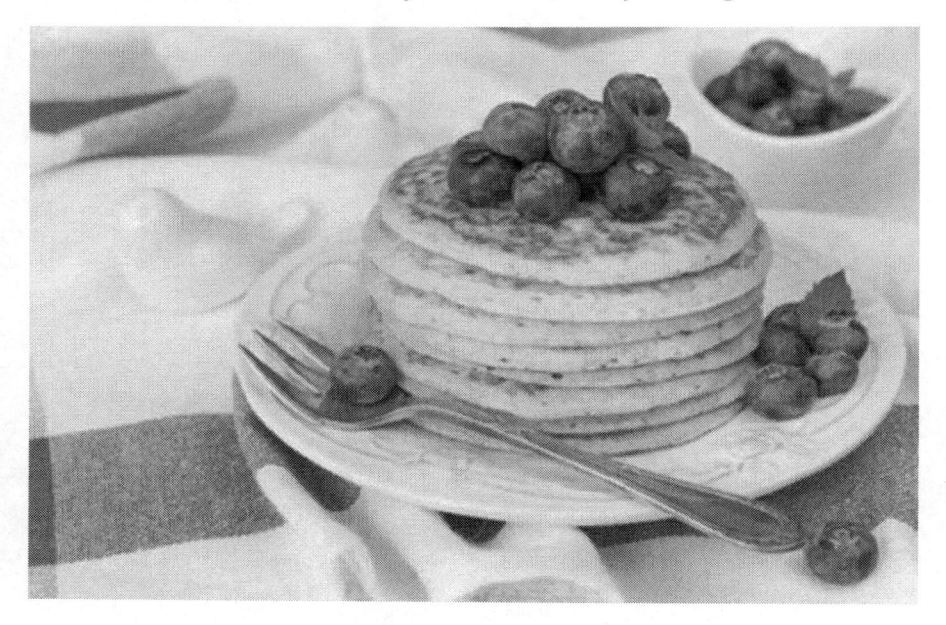

Ingredients:

- 1 cup whole wheat pastry flower
- 1 tablespoon sugar (you can use your preferred type of sugar or sweetener)
- 2 tablespoons baking powder
- 1 dash of sea salt
- 1 cup rice milk
- Blueberries to taste

Instructions:

1. Set out all your ingredients. Place a pan on the stove over medium heat.
2. Combine all your dry ingredients. Add the rice milk to the mixture and beat until smooth.
3. Spoon the mixture onto the pan. When bubbles begin to appear on the surface, flip the pancake over. Cook until it is brown on both sides.
4. Repeat until all the mixture has been used.

Tip: These can be made in large batches and frozen. Just pop them in the microwave when you are ready to eat.

Nutritional Information: 400 calories per serving, 65g carbs, 0g fat, 10g protein, 2.4g fiber

2| French Toast

Servings: 6

Prep Time: 5 Minutes
Cook Time: 10 Minutes

> Who can resist the aroma of French toast? My recipe will allow you to indulge in this classic breakfast dish and not have all the guilt afterwards or spend all morning making them. Fifteen minutes tops! Oh, and as an added bonus...your kids will be looking for seconds.

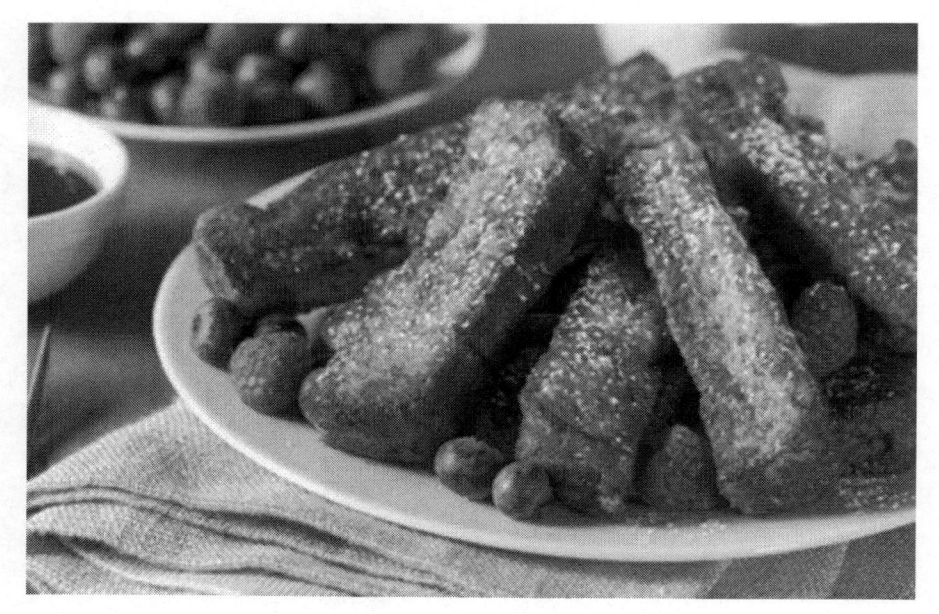

Ingredients:

- 1 cup original almond smooth milk
- ½ cup orange juice
- 2 tablespoons flour
- 1 tablespoon nutritional yeast
- ½ teaspoon cinnamon

- ¼ teaspoon nutmeg
- 6 slices of whole wheat bread

Instructions:

1. Preheat a non-stick skillet over high heat.
2. Add all ingredients to a bowl and mix together.
3. Dip a slice of bread into the mixture and place onto the skillet. Cook for about three minutes on each side.
4. Repeat until you have used all of the mixture and/or bread.
5. Serve and enjoy.

Tip: If you do not use up all of the mixture, you can store it in the fridge for use at a later time. The mixture will keep for up to five days. Also, if you have extra toasts left over, you can always save them to have later on in the day as a snack. All you have to do is toast them. They are great either plain or with a topping such as bananas or peanut butter.

Nutritional Information: 95 calories per serving, 16.6g carbs, 1.1g fat, 4.8g protein, 2.5g fiber

3| Cinnamon Berry Oatmeal

Servings: 2

Prep Time: 5 Minutes
Cook Time: 20 Minutes

> There is nothing more comforting than a nice warm bowl of oatmeal in the morning. This oatmeal is especially wonderful because it is naturally sweet and so healthy.

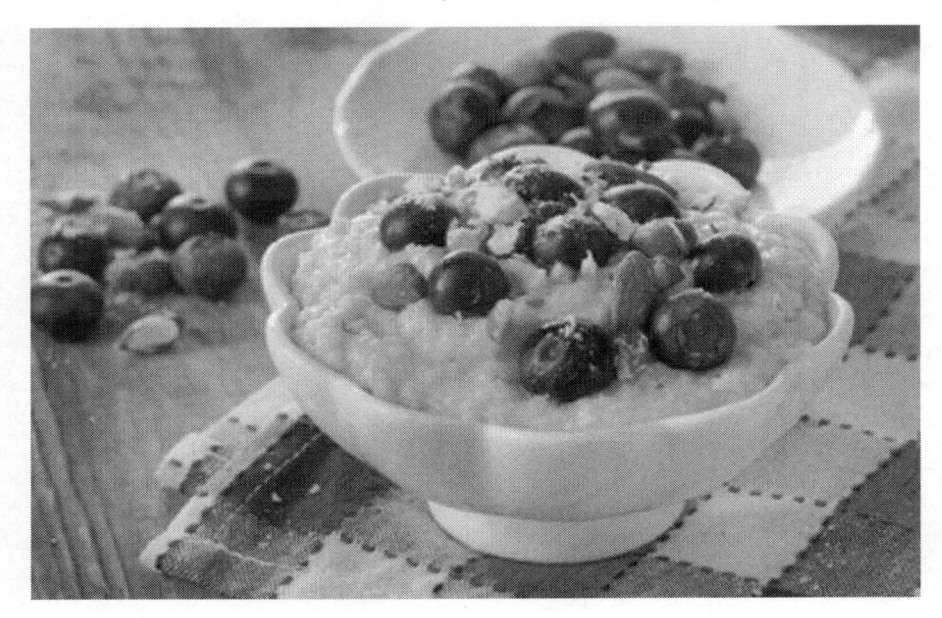

Ingredients:

- 1 cup water
- 1 teaspoon vanilla extract
- 1/4 teaspoon cinnamon
- 1/2 cup old fashioned rolled oats
- 1/2 cup blueberries (fresh or frozen)
- 2 apples, peeled, cored and diced
- 2 teaspoon chopped walnuts or almonds

- 1 tablespoon ground flax seed

Instructions:

1. In a medium saucepan add the water, vanilla and cinnamon and bring to a boil over medium heat.
2. Add the oats and reduce heat to a simmer. Cook for about five minutes.
3. Once the oats have softened, stir in the berries. Continue cooking until all of it is heated through.
4. Remove the saucepan from heat. Cover and let stand 15 minutes or until it reaches the desired thickness. Once the oatmeal has thickened and you are ready to eat, add the apples, nuts and flax.

Nutritional Information: 240.7 calories per serving, 40.8g carbs, 6g fat, 17.7g protein, 6.9g fiber

4| Spicy Southern Grits

Servings: 2

Prep Time: 5 Minutes
Cook Time: 15 Minutes

I have to be totally honest and say that the first time I tried grits, many years ago, I hated them. They were bland and the consistency reminded me of what movies depict as "prison food". It wasn't until recently that I tasted this version of grits that I learned what they are really supposed to look and taste like. I guarantee if you've had a not-so-good grit experience in the past, this will totally change your mind.

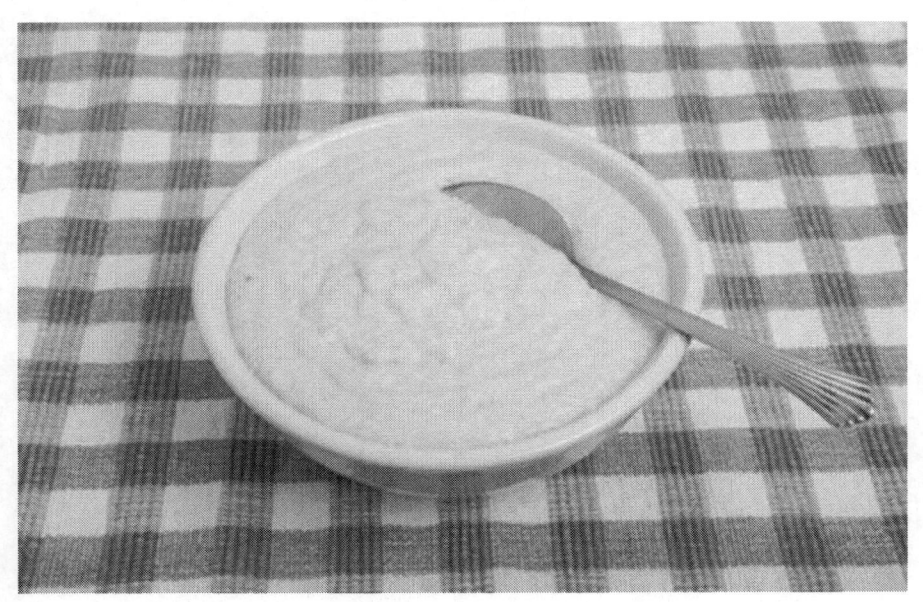

Ingredients:

- 1 small yellow onion, diced
- 1 tablespoon garlic, minced
- ¼ cup green chilies, diced

- 1 chipotle pepper, chopped
- 2 cups veggie stock
- ½ cup grits, yellow
- 3 tablespoons nutritional yeast
- ½ lime, juiced

Instructions:

1. Sautee the onions, garlic, green chilies and chipotle pepper with 2 tablespoons veggie stock for 5 to 7 minutes.
2. Add the rest of the stock and bring to a boil.
3. Using a whisk, add the grits. Turn the heat to low and cook for five minutes.
4. Stir in the nutritional yeast and the limejuice.
5. Once the grits are cooked you can add seasoning to your liking. Serve and enjoy.

Nutritional Information: 137 calories per serving, 24.8g carbs, 3g fat, 9.1g protein, 7.3g fiber

5| Blueberry Muffins

Servings: 1 dozen

Prep Time: 30 Minutes
Cook Time: 30 Minutes

Let's face it. We don't always have the time or desire to sit down and eat breakfast, even if it is the most important meal of the day. Cook up a batch of these muffins ahead of time and have a delicious, quick option you can have on those on-the-go days.

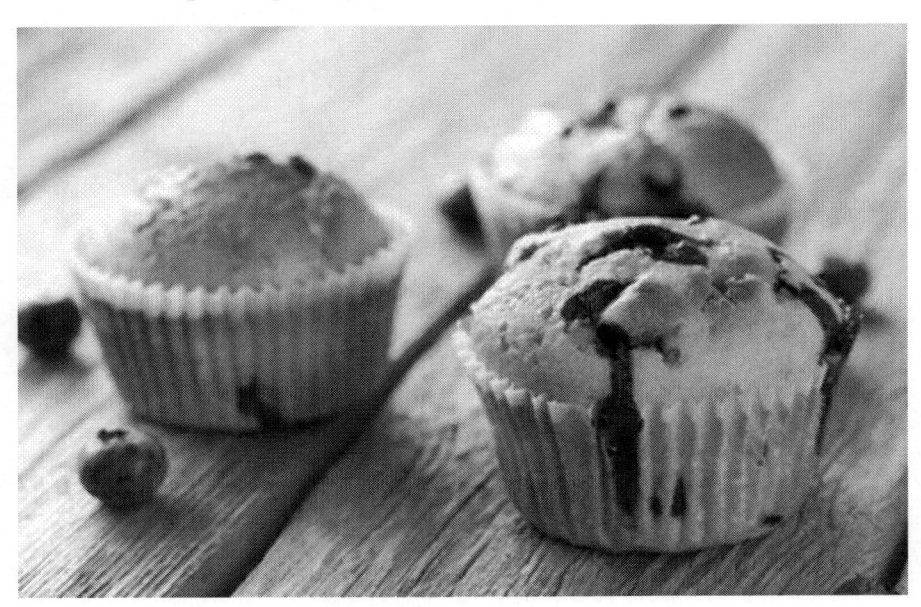

Ingredients:

- 12 dates, pitted and chopped
- 1 cup almond milk
- 1½ cups old-fashioned rolled oats
- ¾ cup dry millet
- 2 teaspoons baking powder
- ½ teaspoon ground cardamom

- ½ cup applesauce
- 1 teaspoon lemon zest, packed
- 1 cup blueberries

Instructions:

1. Preheat your oven to 350. Mix the chopped dates and the almond milk in a small bowl and set aside for about 15 to 20 minutes so that the dates can soften.
2. Using your blender, grind the oats and millet into a flour consistency. Mix the flour, baking powder and cardamom in a separate bowl and stir all the ingredients together.
3. Pour the dates and almond milk mixture into the blender and blend until it is smooth. Add the date mixture to the bowl of dry ingredients along with the applesauce and lemon zest, and mix well until all the dry ingredients have disappeared.
4. Gently fold in the blueberries. Once everything is mixed together, spoon the batter into muffin pan, filling each muffin cup about halfway full.
5. Bake the muffins for 25 to 30 minutes. You will know the muffins are ready when the tops begin to brown and cracks show up on the muffin top. You could also use the "toothpick test" to see if they are ready. Let the muffins cool for at least 15-20 minutes before removing.

Nutritional Information: 129 calories per serving, 19.8g carbs, 5g fat, 2.2g protein, 2.6g fiber

6| Breakfast Cookies

Servings: 12

Prep Time: 10 Minutes
Cook Time: 25 Minutes

So, you've been working hard all week to eat healthy. You deserve a treat, don't you? These breakfast cookies are exactly what you need. They are full of good stuff, so there will be no room for guilt after eating these.

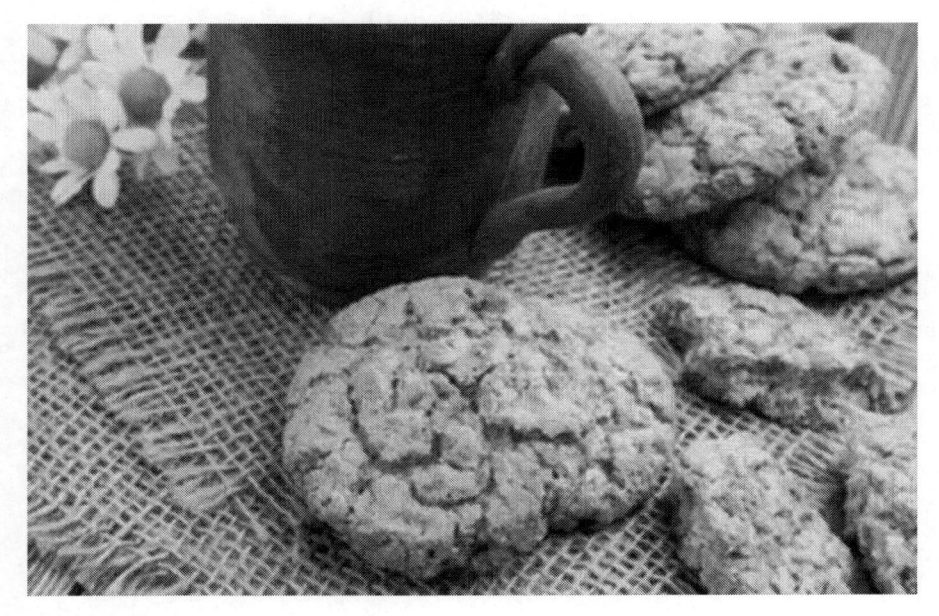

Ingredients:

- ¼ cup unsweetened applesauce
- 2 tablespoons chia seeds
- ½ cup date paste
- 1 teaspoon vanilla extract
- 2 ripe bananas, mashed
- 2 tablespoons fine chopped walnuts
- 1 cup rolled oats
- ½ cup unbleached flour

- ½ teaspoon baking soda

Instructions:

1. Preheat oven to 350 degrees.
2. Combine the applesauce, chia seeds, date paste and vanilla and bananas into a bowl and mix until smooth. Set the bowl aside so that the chia seeds can start to gel.
3. In a separate bowl, combine the walnuts and the dry ingredients. Combine the wet ingredients into this mix. Mix well with a wooden spoon.
4. Scoop the cookies onto the baking sheet. With a spatula or a knife, flatten the cookies to your desired thickness. Thicker cookies will be chewier.
5. Place in oven and bake for 23-25 minutes. Once they are ready, remove and let cool before serving.

Tip: These can be stored in an airtight container or Ziploc and frozen.

Nutritional Information: 92 calories per serving, 18.7g carbs, 1g fat, 2.1g protein, 1.7g fiber

7| Breakfast Tortillas

Servings: 6-8

Prep Time: 10 Minutes
Cook Time: 10 Minutes

Here's a little fancier dish that you can serve occasionally at home, or make for guests. It is very filling and something different to change things up a bit.

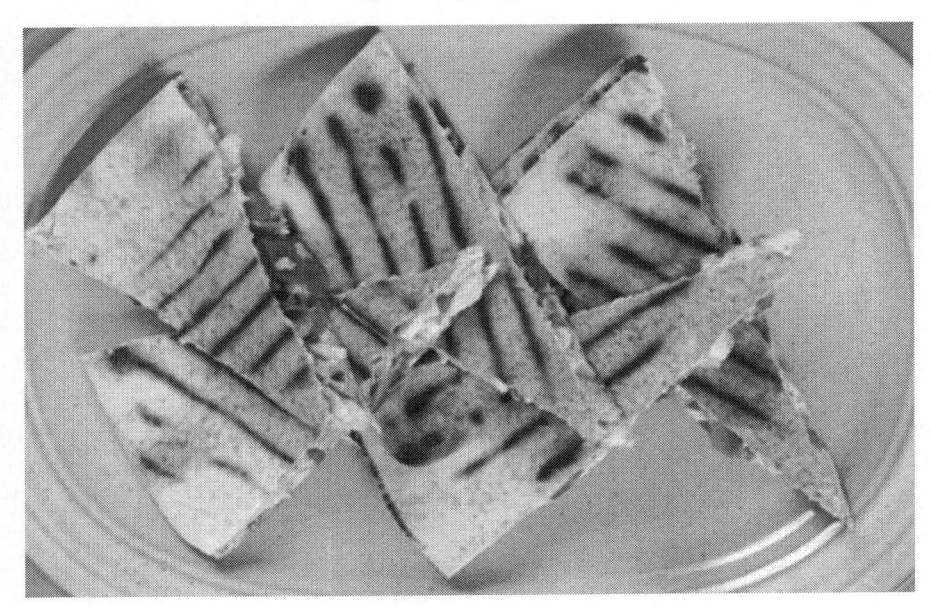

Ingredients:

- 2 cups packed spinach
- 2 cups cooked brown rice
- 1 cup frozen corn kernels
- ½ cup salsa
- 6 to 8 whole wheat or corn tortillas

Instructions:

1. Place the spinach in a saucepan. Make sure that the leaves are wet. Cook for about two minutes, or until it is just wilted. Remove from the saucepan and drain well.
2. Place the brown rice, corn, and salsa in the saucepan. Cook until heated through and then stir in the spinach.
3. Once everything is cooked spoon some of the mixture onto each tortilla and roll.

Nutritional Information: 234 calories per serving, 49.5g carbs, 2g fat, 5.6g protein, 3.7g fiber

Lunch

Recipes Included in this Chapter:

1| Kale, Lemon & Cilantro Sandwich

2| Pesto Pasta

3| Black Bean Tacos

4| Black Beans and Rice

5| Mac n Cheese

6| Black Bean Veggie Burgers

7| Tomato Soup

1| Kale, Lemon & Cilantro Sandwich

Servings: 2-4

Prep Time: 10 Minutes
Cook Time: 5 Minutes

This super easy and quick sandwich will have you licking your fingers. Perfect for a quick lunch that will be very filling and satisfying.

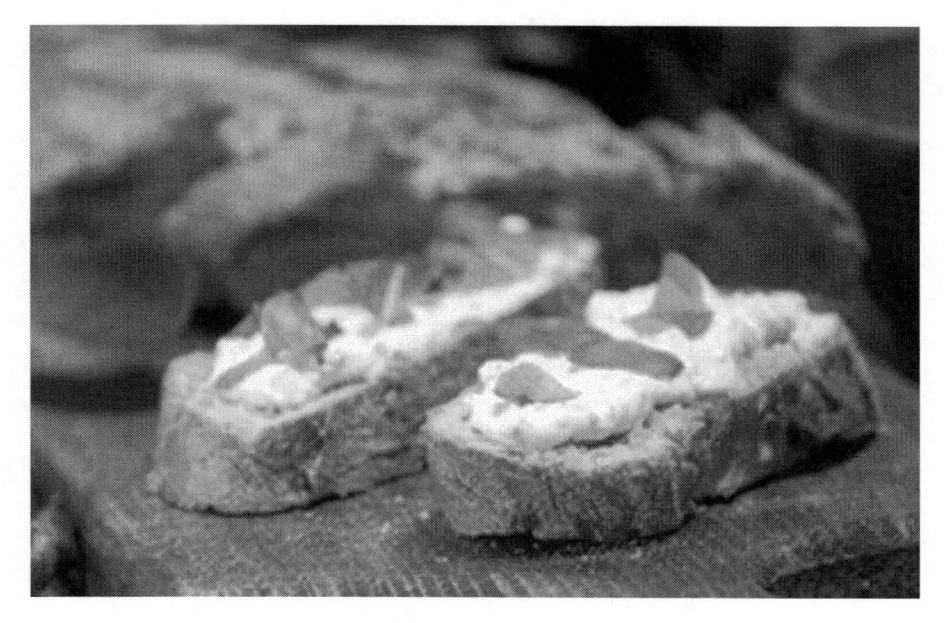

Ingredients:

- 1 bunch kale
- 4 slices whole grain bread
- Hummus
- 4 green onions
- ½ bunch cilantro
- 1 lemon sliced thinly into rounds
- Zest of 1 lemon

Instructions:

1. Tear kale leaves away from thick stem and chop into bite-size pieces. Place the kale in a pot with about 4 inches of water.
2. Bring to a boil, cover and cook until kale is tender. Check frequently.
3. Spread some hummus onto the bread and then add the green onions, cilantro and lemon rounds on top.
4. Once kale is cooked and drained well, sprinkle with the lemon zest. If you really like lemon, you can squeeze the juice of the remaining lemons on also.
5. Place a large handful of the seasoned kale onto the bread and then top with the other slice.

Nutritional Information: 78 calories per serving, 15.3g carbs, 1g fat, 3.8g protein, 2.6g fiber

2| Pesto Pasta

Servings: 4

Prep Time: 5 Minutes
Cook Time: 10 Minutes

> I know what you're thinking — *Don't you need oil and cheese for pesto?* The answer is no! Not for this delicious recipe. Enjoy this light and fresh pasta with some vegetables.

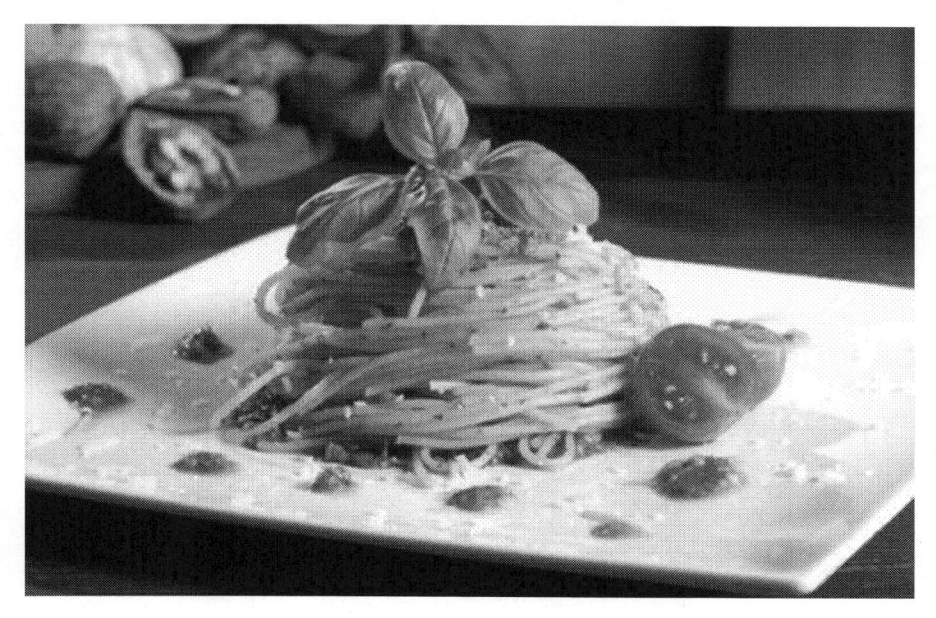

Ingredients:

- ½ cup water
- ½ cup walnuts
- ½ teaspoon minced fresh garlic (1-2 cloves)
- 1 large bunch fresh basil
- 1 package cooked whole-grain pasta of your choice

Instructions:

1. In a food processor, blend all ingredients until smooth. You can use water to thin out as needed.
2. Cook the pasta according to package directions. Once the pasta is cooked, drain.
3. Return the just-cooked pasta to its cooking pot with the heat on medium-low, and add the pesto.
4. Stir until the pasta is completely coated and the pesto is warmed through. Serve while the pesto is still warm.

Nutritional Information: 97 calories per serving, 1.7g carbs, 9g fat, 3.8g protein, 1.1g fiber

3| Black Bean Tacos

Servings: 8

Prep Time: 5 Minutes
Cook Time: 10 Minutes

Who doesn't love a good taco? This recipe will allow you to indulge in some delicious tacos with an amazing cilantro-lime sauce.

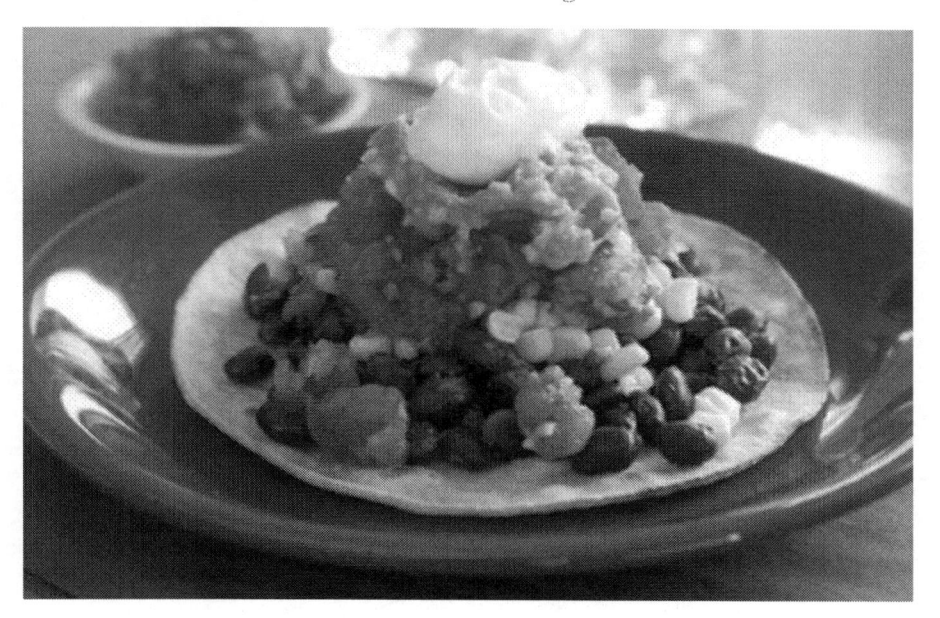

Ingredients:

- 2 cans of black beans
- 1 cup salsa
- 1 teaspoon cumin
- Corn tortillas
- Toppings of your choice
- ½ avocado
- ¾ cup cilantro (leaves only)
- 1 lime, juiced
- 1 garlic clove

- Pinch of salt

Instructions:

1. Begin by preparing the sauce. Add avocado, cilantro, limejuice, garlic and salt to a food processor. Once everything is blended, set aside.
2. Add black beans to a pan over medium heat. Add salsa and cumin. Cook for about five minutes until the beans are heated through.
3. While the beans are heating, warm up your tortillas and prepare your toppings.
4. Assemble your tacos and enjoy!

Nutritional Information: 405 calories per serving, 71g carbs, 4g fat, 24g protein, 17.8g fiber

4| Black Beans and Rice

Servings: 5

Prep Time: 15 Minutes
Cook Time: 10 Minutes

This dish is as basic as they come, but the flavor will tell a whole different story. Prepare this for your family or impress some friends.

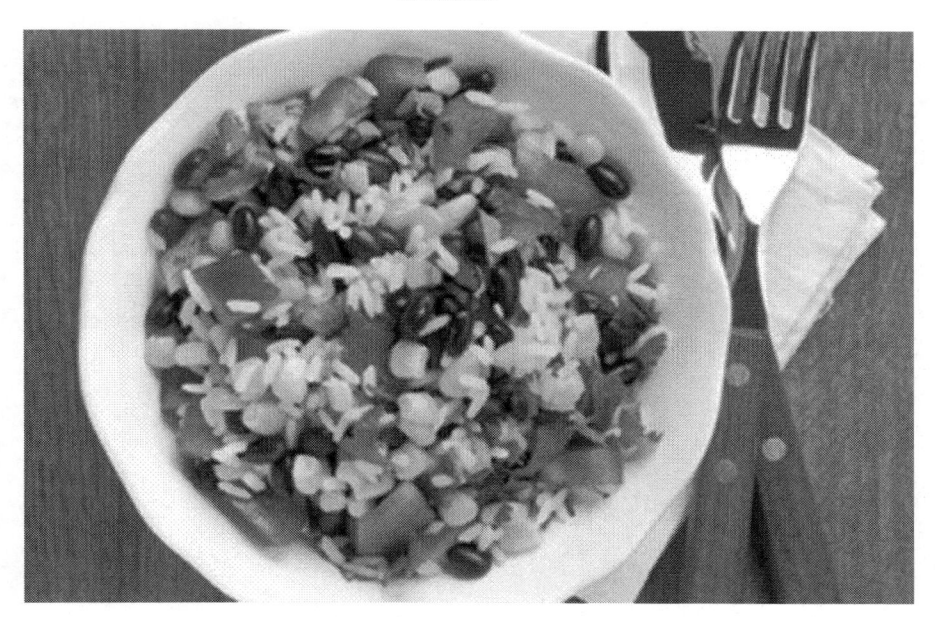

Ingredients:

- 2 cans of black beans
- 1 cup veggie stock
- 1 tablespoon Liquid Aminos
- 1 teaspoon red chili powder
- 2 chopped tomatoes
- 3 chopped green onions
- 1 cup corn
- 2 chopped and seeded green peppers

- 1 bunch cilantro leaves
- 1 avocado
- 3 cups cooked rice
- Salsa to taste

Instructions:

1. Heat the beans with about 2 cups of water, the liquid aminos and chili powder.
2. Serve the rice onto plates. Ladle the beans over the rice according to taste.
3. Add chopped vegetables on top of the rice and beans.
4. Cover with salsa to taste.

Tip: You can use pinto or kidney beans in place of black beans.

Nutritional Information: 703 calories per serving, 119g carbs, 10g fat, 39g protein, 30.3g fiber

5| Mac n' Cheese

Servings: 6

Prep Time: 20 Minutes
Cook Time: 20 Minutes

Nothing says all-American like a nice warm bowl of Mac n' Cheese. Well, now even us Vegans can enjoy this all-time favorite.

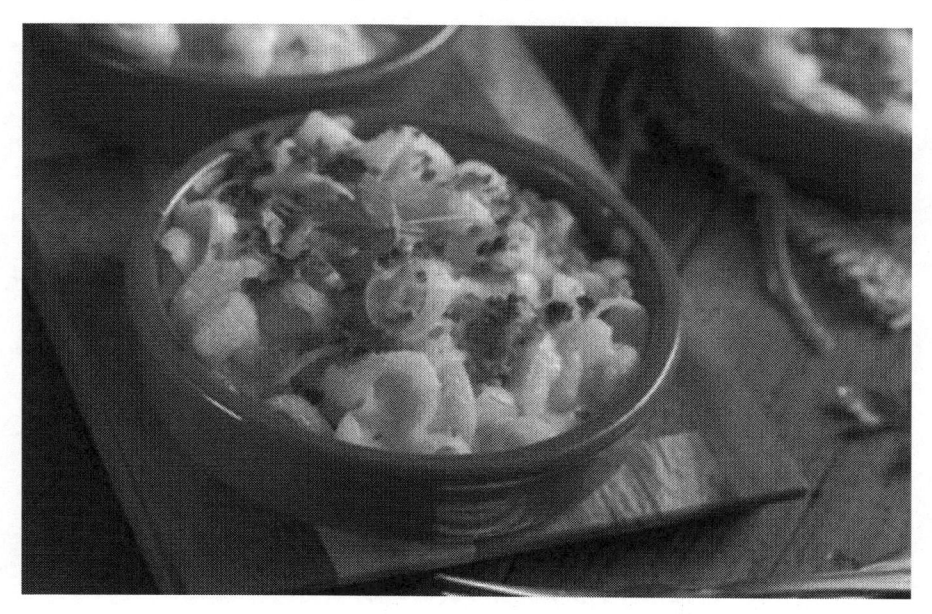

Ingredients:

- 1½ cups raw cashews
- 3 tablespoons lemon juice
- ¾ cup water
- 1½ teaspoon sea salt
- ¼ cup nutritional yeast
- ½ teaspoon chili powder
- ½ clove garlic
- pinch of turmeric
- pinch of cayenne pepper
- ½ teaspoon Dijon mustard

- 8 oz. of elbow or shell pasta of choice

Instructions:

1. Preheat the oven to 350F. Start boiling some water to prepare your pasta. Cook according to package directions.
2. Add the cashews into a blender and blend until they are finely ground. Once the cashews have been processed and are the correct consistency, add the rest of the ingredients and blend until you have a thick smooth consistency.
3. By this point, your pasta should be ready or very close to it. Once it is cooked to your liking, drain and rinse it. Once drained, return it to the pot. Now add the "cheese sauce" and mix well with the pasta. Let it sit on low heat for a couple of minutes to heat the sauce through.
4. Serve while hot and enjoy!

Tip: *You can also add veggies to this dish. Some delish sautéed broccoli would make this dish even more amazing.*

Nutritional Information: 224 calories per serving, 14.7g carbs, 10g fat, 8.4g protein, 2.9g fiber

6| Black Bean Veggie Burger

Servings: 6

Prep Time: 15 Minutes
Cook Time: 35 Minutes

I'm sure you would agree that no collection of vegan recipes would be complete without a vegan burger recipe. Well, here we are giving you a great burger you can cook up in no time.

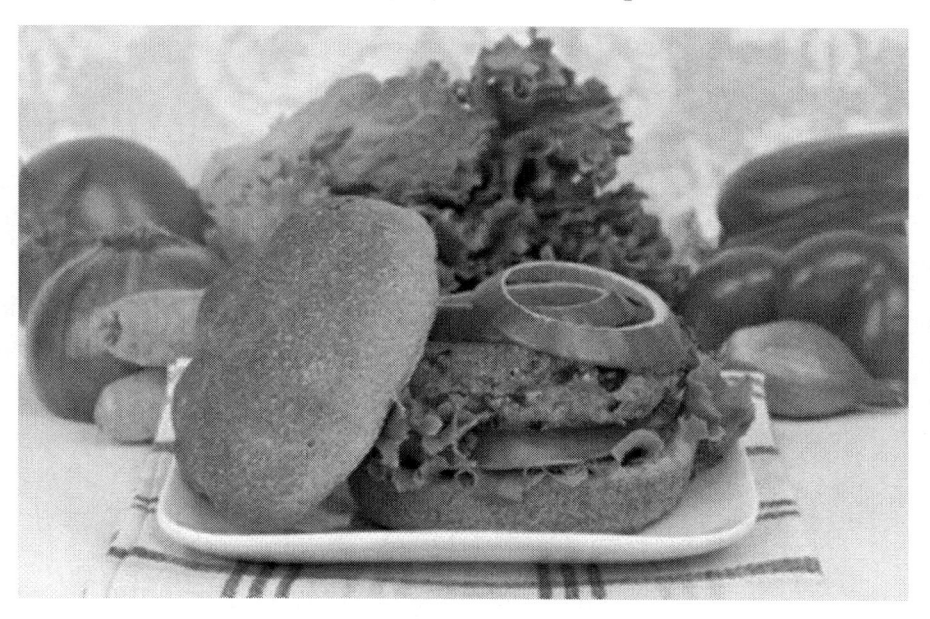

Ingredients:

- 1 red bell pepper
- 5 small red potatoes
- 2 cans black beans, drained and rinsed
- ¾ cup smooth salsa
- 2 teaspoons chili powder
- 1 teaspoon ground cumin
- ¼ cup medium grind coarse cornmeal

Instructions:

1. Preheat oven to 400 degrees.
2. Chop your bell pepper. Make sure to cut it into small pieces so that it will mix easily with the burger batter. Place them onto a sheet pan lined with parchment paper and roast in the oven for about 10 minutes.
3. Peel the potatoes and wrap them in plastic. Cook them in the microwave until they are tender. Alternately, you could roast them, but do NOT boil as boiling will make the burgers mushy. Mash the cooked potatoes and measure out 1 tightly packed cup. Set this aside.
4. Drain and rinse your black beans. Make sure there is no excess water on the beans. Measure out 1 cup of the black beans and place into a large mixing bowl. The rest of the beans should be placed into a food processor. Add the potatoes to the processor as well. Pulse until you have a sticky, thick mashed paste. It should only take a few pulses.
5. Add this mixture to the bowl of extra beans.
6. In a separate small bowl, combine the salsa, chili powder, and cumin and mix well. Pour the salsa mixture over the bowl of beans and potatoes and add the cooked bell pepper.
7. Mix all of the ingredients together until everything is combined well and you have a thick, sticky paste.
8. Lastly, mix the cornmeal into the batter until combined well. Place the batter into the fridge for 30 minutes prior to baking. This will help with forming the patties later on.
9. After chilling, form 6 patties and place them on a sheet pan lined with parchment paper.
10. Bake at 375 degrees for 25 minutes. Remove the pan and using a thin metal spatula carefully flip them. After you have flipped all 6 patties, cook for additional 10 minutes.
11. Remove the patties from the oven and let cool while you prepare your patties and the toppings you will use.

Nutritional Information: 616 calories per serving, 117.6g carbs, 2.7g fat, 34g protein, 25.6g fiber

7| Tomato Soup

Servings: varies depending on use

Prep Time: 20 Minutes
Cook Time: 20 Minutes

> To round up our delicious lunch section, we are offering you a wonderful and easy-to-prepare soup. This soup is great year round.

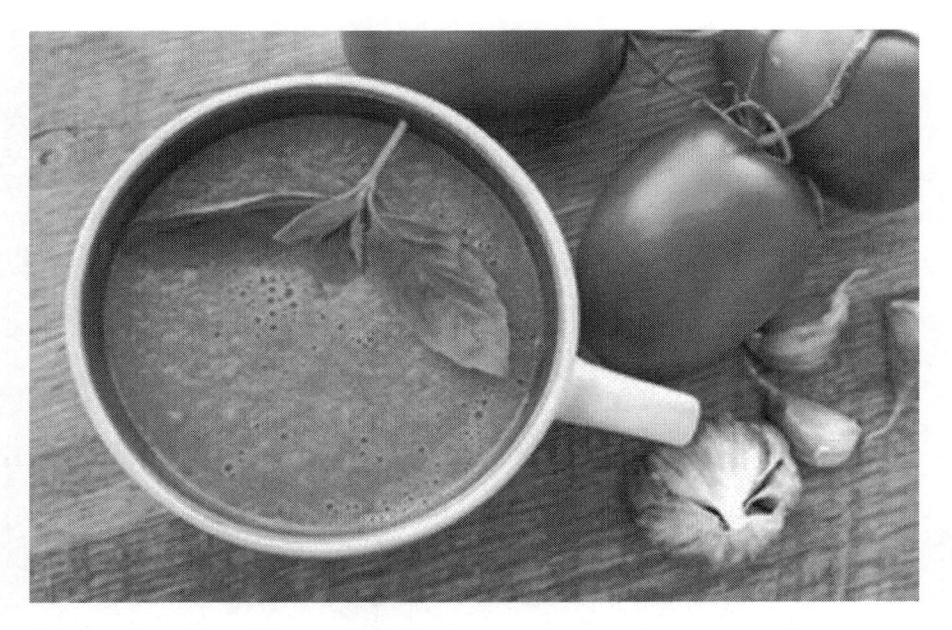

Ingredients:

- 1 onion, diced
- 2 garlic cloves, minced
- 2 tablespoons water
- 4 lbs. ripe tomatoes
- 1 cup vegetable broth
- Cilantro for garnish

Instructions:

1. Prepare a large pot with water and add the diced onion and minced garlic. Cook until they are soft, adding water as necessary.
2. Add the tomatoes (which should be peeled, seeded, and chopped) and broth to the pot. Bring to a boil then reduce heat and simmer for about 15 minutes.
3. Once this is cooked, add to a blender and puree.
4. Serve the soup and garnish with some cilantro or other herb of your choosing.

Nutritional Information: 139 calories per serving, 27.9g carbs, 1.7g fat, 7.5g protein, 8.1g fiber

Dinner

Recipes Included in this Chapter:

1| Black Bean Wrap

2| Quinoa Teriyaki

3| Shepard's Pie

4| Vegetable Pasta

5| Lasagna Rolls

6| Tortilla Casserole

7| Chickpea Chili

1| Black Bean Wrap

Servings: 1

Prep Time: 5 Minutes
Cook Time: 5 Minutes

Let's face it. We don't always want a big elaborate production when it comes to dinner. This wrap will help you serve a dish that is filling and tastes great without all the fuss.

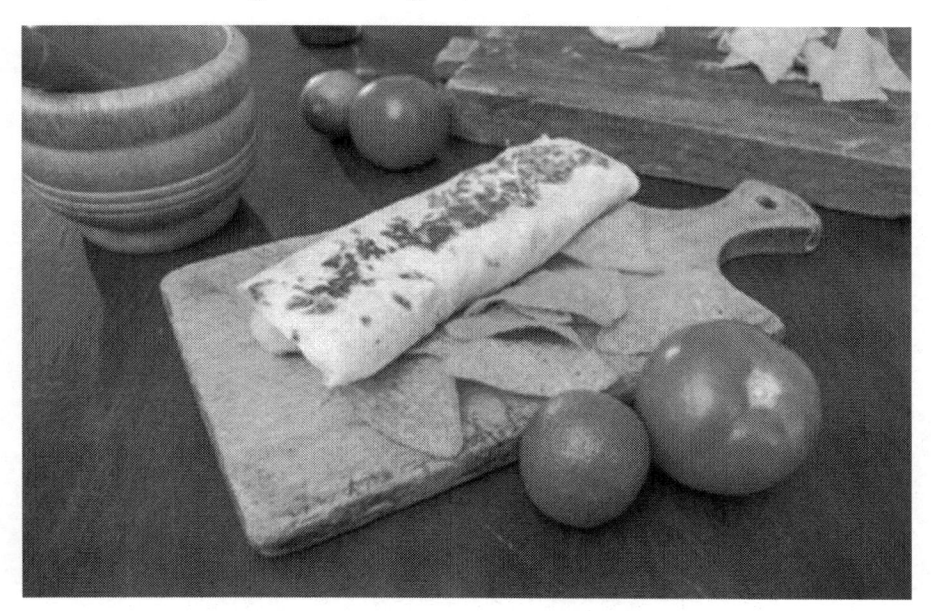

Ingredients:

- 1 large whole grain tortilla
- ⅓ cup salsa
- ¼ cup black beans
- ¼ cup corn
- ¼ avocado, chopped
- 1 large handful of baby greens
- 2 sprigs of cilantro, chopped

Instructions:

1. Warm tortilla using your preferred method.
2. Pour salsa onto the tortilla. It's best to keep to one side in order to make the wrapping part easier.
3. Spread the black beans, corn, and avocado over salsa.
4. Sprinkle the cilantro over the bean mixture and then top with the greens of your choosing.
5. Fold sides of the wrap over the ingredients and then roll from one side to the other. Cut the wrap in half and serve.

Nutritional Information: 269 calories per serving, 34.7g carbs, 10g fat, 11g protein, 10g fiber

2| Quinoa Teriyaki

Servings: 4

Prep Time: 5 Minutes
Cook Time: 10 Minutes

This dish is satisfying and the texture of it is amazing. It's chewy and creamy all in one. It'll be a hit at the dinner table.

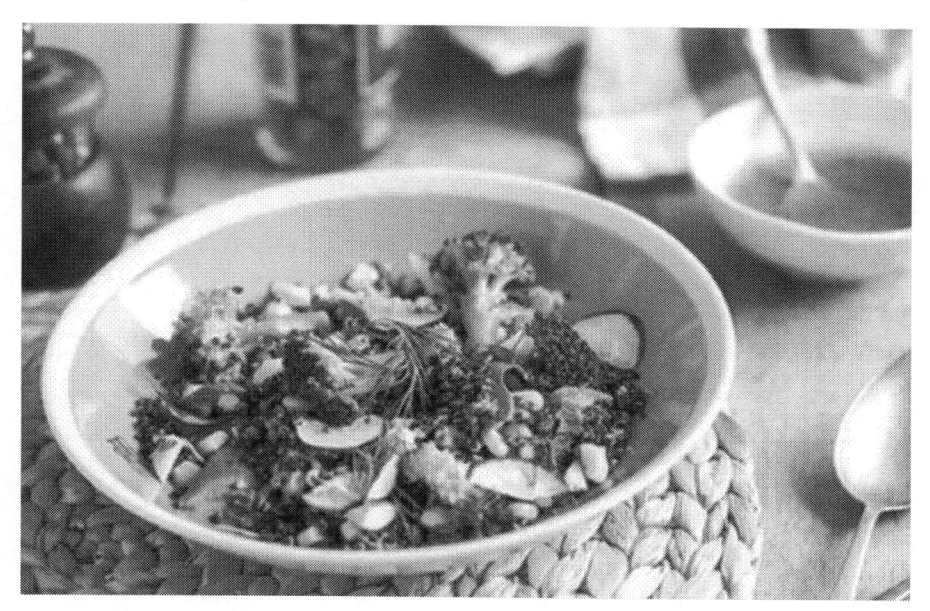

Ingredients:

- 2 large baked sweet potatoes
- 2 cups cooked quinoa
- ¼ cup water
- 4 cups broccoli florets
- 1 small onion
- 1 avocado
- ½ cup teriyaki sauce

Instructions:

1. Add ¼ cup of water to a sauté pan. Add chopped onion, mushrooms and broccoli. Cover and cook on medium high heat for about 10 minutes. Stir occasionally.
2. Warm up the quinoa and sweet potatoes separately in the microwave.
3. When the vegetables are done, add the warmed up quinoa to the sauté pan and stir to mix with vegetables.
4. Serve warmed sweet potatoes into bowls according to servings.
5. Add the quinoa/vegetable mixture right atop of the sweet potatoes and then cover with avocados.
6. Drizzle teriyaki sauce according to taste. Mix lightly and enjoy.

Nutritional Information: 486 calories per serving, 72g carbs, 10g fat, 18g protein, 12g fiber

3| Shepard's Pie

Servings: 6

Prep Time: 35 Minutes
Cook Time: 60 Minutes

> This Shepard's pie recipe makes me reminisce of my childhood and when I would sit at the table with my family. Create a new memory for your family or friends with the healthy vegan dish.

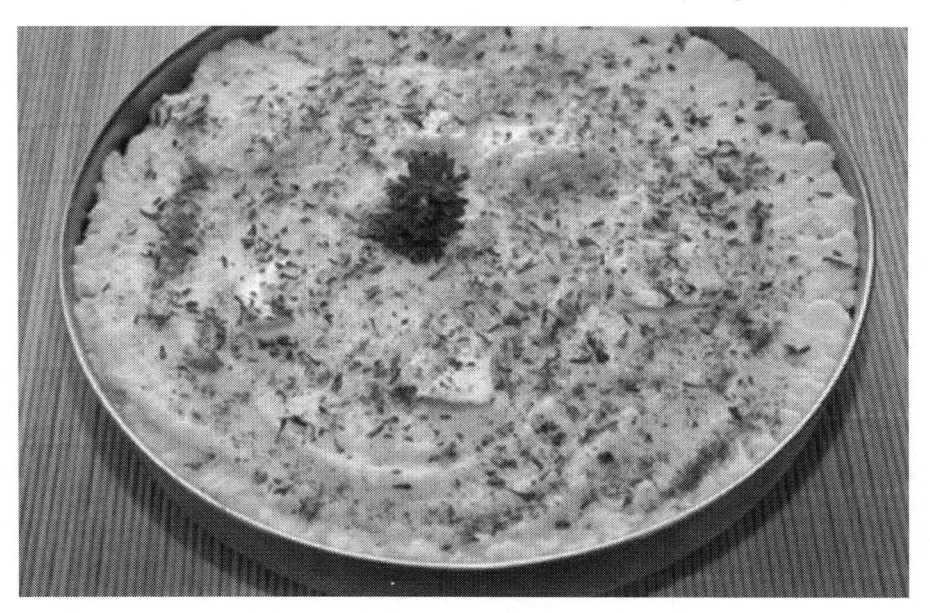

Ingredients:

- 3 cups veggie broth
- 1 chopped onion
- 1 celery stalk
- 1 green pepper
- ½ teaspoon sage leaves
- 1 tablespoon soy sauce
- 1 carrot
- 1 ½ cups cauliflower florets

- 1 cup cabbage
- 1 cup greens beans
- mix of 2 tablespoons cornstarch & 1/3 cup cold water
- pepper to taste
- 3 cups mashed potatoes

Instructions:

1. Preheat oven to 350F.
2. In a large pot, cook ½ cup veggie broth, onion, celery, bell pepper and garlic. Make sure to stir occasionally, for about 4 minutes. Add the sage and soy sauce and stir. Then add the remaining vegetable broth along with the carrots, cauliflower, cabbage and green beans.
3. Bring to a boil and cover, then reduce heat and cook for 20 minutes on low-medium heat.
4. Add the cornstarch mixture and stir until it begins to thicken. Season with pepper to taste.
5. Transfer to a casserole dish and cover vegetable mixture with mashed potatoes. Bake for 30 minutes or until potatoes are slightly browned.

Nutritional Information: 127 calories per serving, 25.5g carbs, 1.6g fat, 4g protein, 2g fiber

4| Vegetable Pasta

Servings: 4-6

Prep Time: 15 Minutes
Cook Time: 15 Minutes

This one-pot pasta recipe will be the recipe that will keep on giving. Why? Substitute different vegetables and pasta sauce every time you make it and will be like a whole new dish each time.

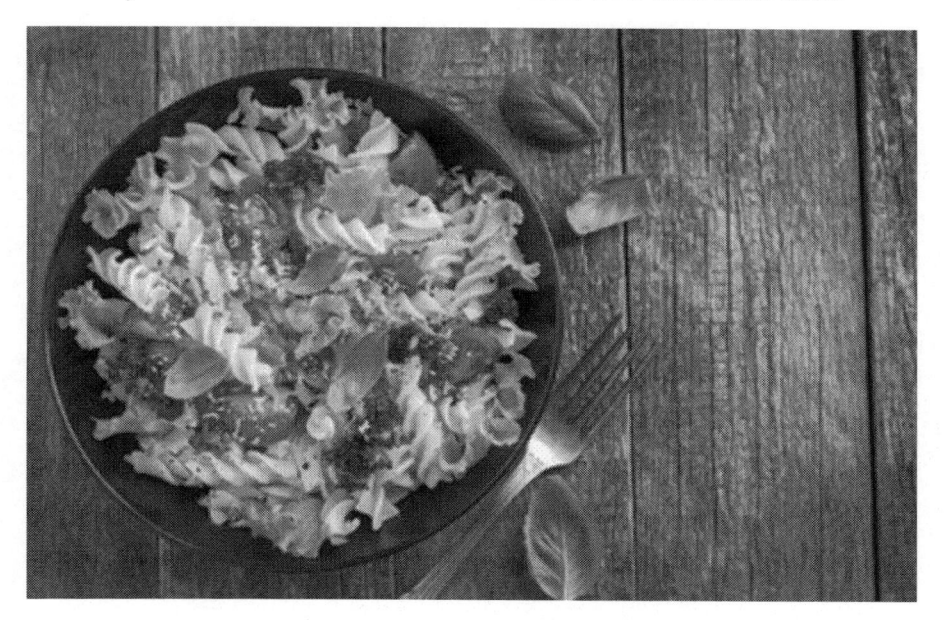

Ingredients:

- 1 lb. pasta (preferably wholegrain)
- 2 cups broccoli florets
- bunch of spinach
- cherry tomatoes
- 1 jar of your favorite pasta sauce

Instructions:

1. Cook pasta in a large pot according to package directions.
2. In a separate pot, cook vegetables according to preferred softness.
3. Drain the pasta and vegetables then add everything into one pot and mix with pasta sauce.

Nutritional Information: 245 calories per serving, 46.2g carbs, 2g fat, 11g protein, 2g fiber

5| Lasagna Rolls

Servings: 5

Prep Time: 10 Minutes
Cook Time: 25 Minutes

Lasagna is one of my favorite dinner dishes. It's great for dinner parties or for a few guests. Cook up a batch and serve this at your next get-together or for a simple family meal.

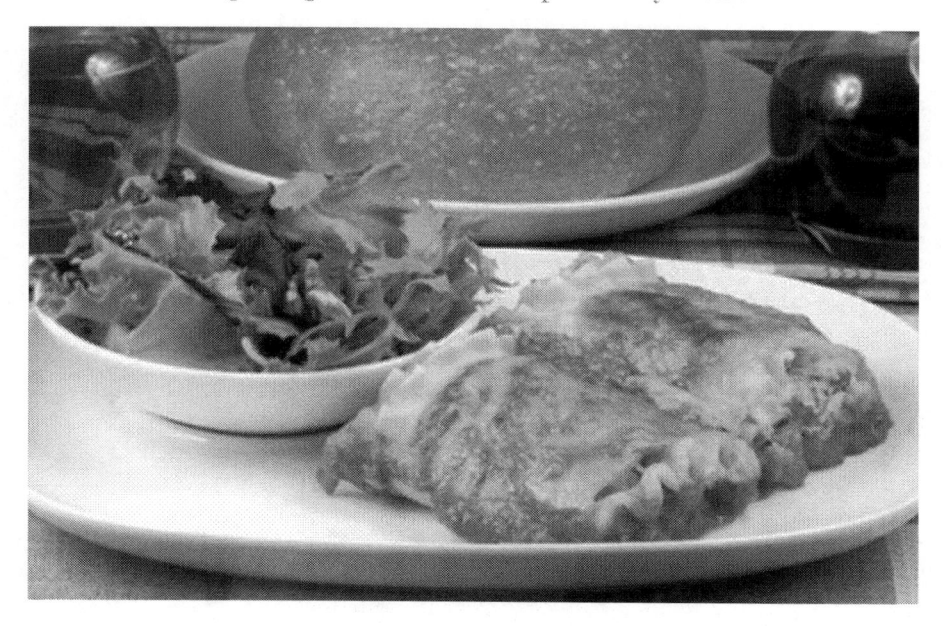

Ingredients:

- lasagna noodles
- 2 ripe avocados
- 2 tablespoons vegan Parmesan
- ¼ teaspoon garlic powder
- 2 teaspoon basil
- 1/3 cup chopped baby spinach leaves
- 1 tablespoon parsley
- 6 grape tomatoes

- pepper to taste
- ½ cup sauce

Instructions:

1. Preheat oven to 350F.
2. Cook about 5 lasagna noodles according to package directions.
3. Combine to avocado, Parmesan, garlic powder, basil, spinach, parsley, tomatoes and pepper. Mix all these ingredients until they are well combined.
4. In a baking dish, cover the bottom with marinara sauce.
5. Take one lasagna noodle and place it on a clean flat surface. Spread some of the mixture across the entire length of the noodle. Roll up the noodle and place upright into the baking dish. Repeat this for all the noodles.
6. Cover the dish with aluminum foil and bake for 20 minutes.

Nutritional Information: 281 calories per serving, 23g carbs, 17g fat, 5g protein, 9g fiber

6| Tortilla Casserole

Servings: 6

Prep Time: 15 Minutes
Cook Time: 15 Minutes

This casserole is a one-dish wonder. You can have dinner ready on the table in 30 minutes! Great for those long days.

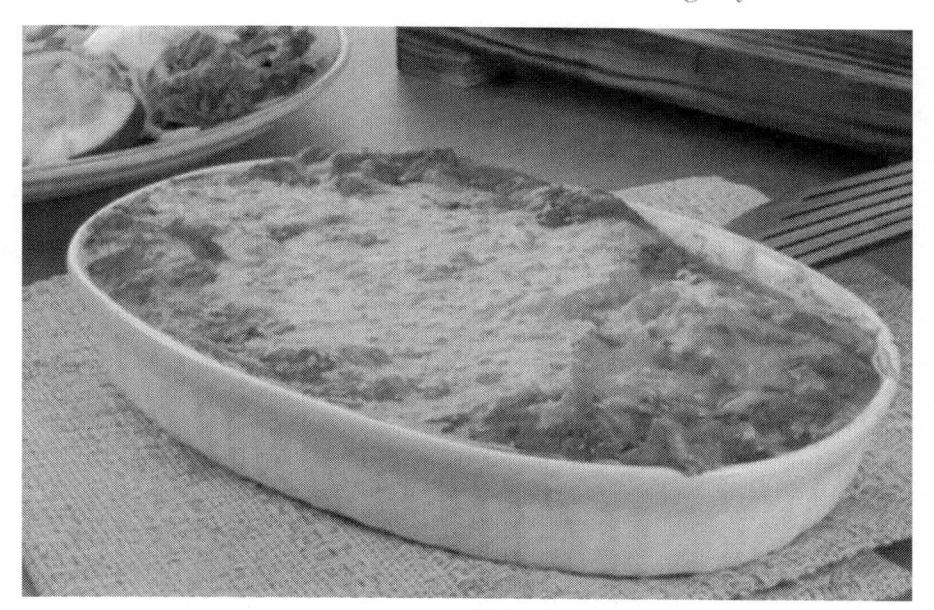

Ingredients:

- 1 can black beans, drained and rinsed
- 1 can diced tomatoes
- 1 can chopped mild green chilies
- 2 cups corn kernels
- 1 bunch scallions, chopped
- 1 teaspoon chili powder
- 1 teaspoon ground cumin
- ½ teaspoon dried oregano

- 12 corn tortillas
- 2 cups vegan cheese
- Salsa

Instructions:

1. Preheat oven to 400° F.
2. Combine beans, tomatoes, chilies, corn, scallions, chili powder, cumin, and oregano in a bowl.
3. Line the bottom of a casserole dish with 6 tortillas, allowing them to overlap in the middle. Scoop on half of the bean mixture and sprinkle on half of the cheese. Add another layer of tortillas as you did before and add the rest of the bean mixture and the rest of the cheese.
4. Bake in the oven for 12-15 minutes.
5. Cut into squares and serve with your favorite salsa.

Nutritional Information: 396 calories per serving, 77g carbs, 2.9g fat, 19g protein, 15.6g fiber

7| Chickpea Chili

Servings: 6

Prep Time: 35 Minutes
Cook Time: 45 Minutes

This chili is a great comfort dish everyone will love. It will be worth the wait, guaranteed.

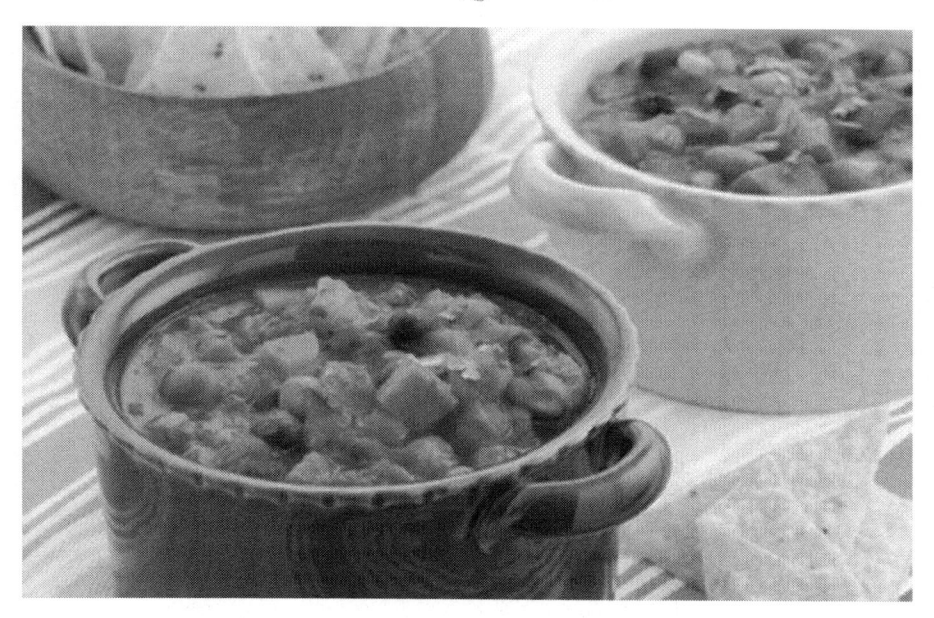

Ingredients:

- 1 diced onion
- 2 garlic cloves, minced
- 1 diced jalapeño
- 2 cans chickpeas
- 1 can of creamy white bean of choice
- 1 can diced green chiles (=chilies)
- 1½ teaspoon cumin
- 1 teaspoon dried thyme
- ¼ teaspoon pepper

- 1 teaspoon oregano
- 1 teaspoon smoked paprika
- 1 teaspoon chili powder
- 3 cups vegetable stock
- 1 cup corn

Instructions:

1. In a pot sauté the onion, garlic and jalapeño over medium heat for 5 minutes.
2. Add the beans, diced green chiles and all the spices. Mix everything well. Stir in the broth and simmer for 20-30 minutes.
3. Add the corn and let simmer for about 2-3 minutes longer.
4. Serve hot with your favorite toppings.

Nutritional Information: 35 calories per serving, 8g carbs, 0.5g fat, 1.2g protein, 1.5g fiber

Snacks

Recipes Included in this Chapter:

1| *Vanilla Chia Pudding*

2| *Baked Sweet Potato Chips*

1| Vanilla Chia Pudding

Servings: 2

Prep Time: 5 Minutes
Cook Time: 5 Minutes

This recipe will take you a total of ten minutes to prepare ahead of time. Have in your fridge to enjoy a smooth, delicious pudding when a snack attack strikes.

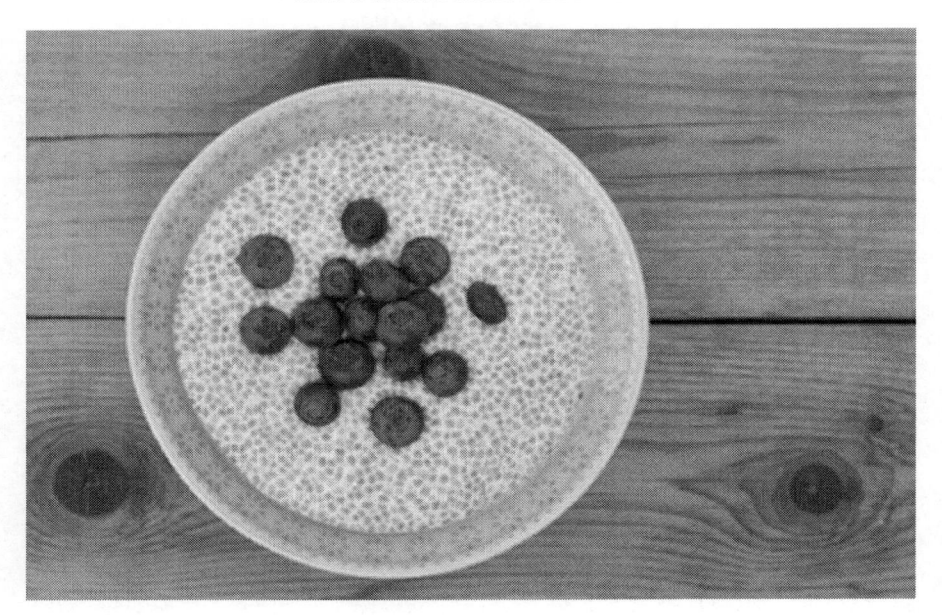

Ingredients:

- 1 cup Rice Milk
- 4 tablespoons chia seeds
- ½ teaspoon vanilla extract

Instructions:

1. Place all of your ingredients into a jar or container that can be shaken.
2. Shake well then place in the refrigerator for at least an hour or overnight.
3. Enjoy.

Nutritional Information: 63 calories per serving, 12.6g carbs, 1g fat, 0g protein, 0g fiber

2| Baked Sweet Potato Chips

Servings: 1-2

Prep Time: 15 Minutes
Cook Time: 12 Minutes

The perfect snack! These oil-free and easy to prepare chips will be just what you need to satisfy your craving for salty and crunchy.

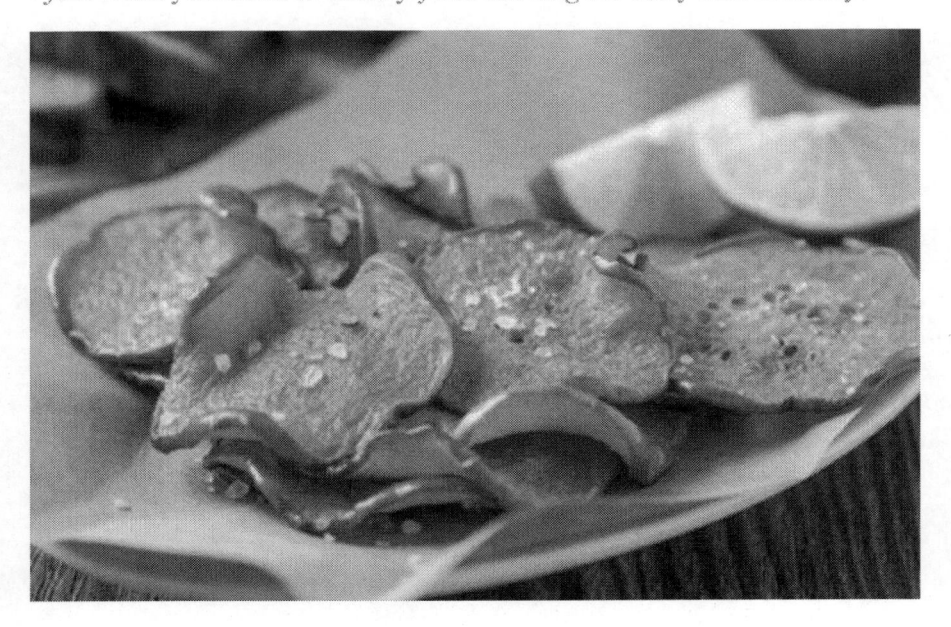

Ingredients:

- Large sweet potato
- Fine sea salt, to taste
- Seasonings of choice

Instructions:

1. Preheat oven to 400F.
2. Slice the potato into really thin slices, with or without the skin. (The use of a mandolin will be your best option, but it is not the only option.)
3. Prepare a baking sheet lined with parchment paper and arrange the slices in a single layer.
4. Sprinkle with sea salt and any other seasoning you have chosen.
5. Bake in the oven for 10 minutes. Flip each slice and continue to bake for another 2-3 minutes. Make sure to keep an eye on them because they will burn easily.

Nutritional Information: 163 calories per serving, 37.3g carbs, 0.3g fat, 3.6g protein, 6g fiber

Final Thoughts

Reversing diabetes is not impossible! You can do it. It will take some changes in the way you are eating, but these changes will give you your life back! So any change that gives you your life back is well worth it.

Changes to your body are going to take time and it is important for you to understand this and stick with this program. Slowly starting to eat more vegetables and other vegan foods will make you feel better and you can start decreasing the other foods that you are eating.

Diabetes is a debilitating disease that can overwhelm you with symptoms and make it difficult to overcome. But you are strong enough to overcome this! You are dedicated and have the strength to regain your health. It is your dedication that is making the reversal of diabetes possible. You have the strength that you have always dreamed of to truly take control of your health.

Think about all the problems that diabetes has brought into your life. By eating a starch-based, vegan, low-fat diet you will be able to combat those negative events. You will start to see changes in how your body processes foods and how you relate to foods. Those problems are about to disappear as you reverse diabetes forever. You will not have to deal with any of those issues ever again.

No longer will you have to have blurred vision or headaches because of your high blood sugars. You will not have to feel those terrible lows when your blood sugars decline. This program will forever change your body and your health.

Starting any new program is overwhelming, but changing to a vegan lifestyle can seem especially hard. Many people struggle to give up animal products and their body craves them. But as you start eating more and more healthy vegan foods your body will not crave the bad food as much.

You will see changes in how your whole body looks and feels while you are going through this process of reversing diabetes. Slowly, you will see the negative problems you have developed from diabetes start to disappear and in their place you will see more positives in your life.

Any change that you make to your life will take time to impliment. So give yourself plenty of time to get used to all the changes you are making to your eating. It is all right if you do not feel comfortable yet, you soon will feel great!

By changing your diet to a nutrient-rich, low-fat, vegan diet, you will be able to fill your body with the best fuel to keep your body functioning at its peak. Your body will be able to process foods better, manage sugar levels better, and burn off fat faster.

Diets of every kind have been started and stopped by people all around the world. But this program is not a diet. This is a scientifically-proven way to feel better and eat a better diet to help reverse your diabetes. When you eat a vegan diet you are committing to being healthier in every aspect of your life. Through this program you will get your blood sugar levels healthy, but you will also get your blood pressure, weight, cholesterol and many other health issues under control.

It is amazing how many physical ailments can be traced back to the type of diet a person is eating. You will be a great example to all those around you about the benefits of a vegan low-fat diet and how it can make your overall health so much better. Research has proven that people who eat a vegan diet have many fewer health concerns.

So why wouldn't anyone want to have better health? The truth is, it can be very overwhelming to change an eating pattern that someone has spent their entire life developing. You will come across obstacles in this process and it will be your inner strength that gets you through it.

No matter what, do not give up. Keep taking it one day at a time as you battle to reverse your diabetes. This program is not easy, but it is worth it. Your health is worth it! You living to be there for your children is worth it. Even if there are days when you are not able to stick to the vegan diet, get back focused for the next day.

Eating a vegan diet is better for your health than any other way of eating. Using vegetables as your main source of food is going to give you a high volume of vitamins and minerals with every meal. These nutrients will help your hair, nails, skin and whole body look better and feel better than you can ever imagine.

Use the list of vegan foods to help you plan your meals and choose healthy snacks that are rich in protein. Keeping a balanced diet that is rich in protein will help your body process sugars better and push your body to function at its peak.

Visiting with your doctor on a regular basis is also very important and will help you understand the changes your body is making.

Your doctor can help you make medication changes as needed and build on the success you are already having.

As your health changes you will start to feel more and more comfortable talking about the eating changes you have made. Many of your friends and family that were not supportive in the beginning will start coming around and asking what you are doing to make yourself look so great.

Share your knowledge about the vegan low-fat diet that is working for you. Your friends and family have seen you make this change and they will want to try it for themselves. If you feel comfortable, even show them your journal to see how your blood sugar levels have changed throughout this process and how the other body changes have affected you.

You are an inspiration to those around you! Many of your friends and family will want to imitate you now that they see what you are doing is actually working.

Use your journal to keep track of your eating and blood sugars and show your journal to your doctor to help them make medication changes as you go through the process of reversing your diabetes!

More groundbreaking studies

Don't miss Dr. John McDougalls new FREE Webinars. Dr. John McDougall shares how he treats and helps his patients revert diabetes with diet:

Part 1

www.youtube.com/watch?v=6u4IiVbPdKk

Part 2

www.youtube.com/watch?v=WGPO5Fg8_4s

More free webinars at: www.drmcdougall.com/webinars

Dr. Barnard's clinical studies:

www.nealbarnard.org

Dr. Barnard's groundbreaking clinical studies, the latest funded by the National Institutes of Health, show that diabetes responds dramatically to a low-fat, vegetarian diet. Rather than just compensating for malfunctioning insulin like other treatment plans, Dr. Barnard's program helps repair how the body uses insulin.[6]

---

[6] Neal Barnard, MD, "Dr. Neal Barnard's Program for Reversing Diabetes," n.d., http://www.pcrm.org/shop/byNealBarnard/dr-barnards-program-for-reversing-diabetes.

NEW: Your Body, Your Friend

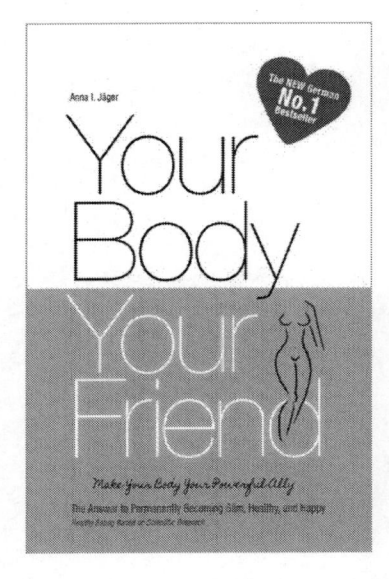

The NEW German No. 1 Bestseller: Your Body, Your Friend

The Answer to Permanently Becoming Slim, Healthy, and Happy
Based on Scientific Research

Fat Storer Goodbye!
Fat Burner Hello.

In the course of her research, bestselling author and long-time nutritionist Anna I. Jäger discovered a fairly simple, logical solution: We need to stop fighting against the biologically natural processes of the organism that we call our bodies. We need to, instead, join forces with them! A healthy, well-nourished body will run more efficiently and lose its extra pounds automatically.

No, these are not false promises; this is biology.

Your Body Needs Energy to Heal
Your Body Needs Energy to Feel Happy
Your Body Needs Energy to Burn Fat (!)

As you read through these chapters, you'll learn:

- How to train your body to become a fat burner, not a fat storer
- Why cutting calories is dangerous for your mind and body
- Why low carb diets will make you gain more fat longterm
- How to overcome an eating disorder
- How to lower your set-point (the weight your body tries to maintain)

Make Your Body Your Powerful Ally

Get this book so you can learn how you can transform your body and life starting today by becoming best friends with your body and nourishing yourself into a new, slim, healthy, and happy you!

ISBN-13: 978-1508525448
ISBN-10: 1508525447

Famous Dishes Made VEGAN!

Famous Dishes Made VEGAN!

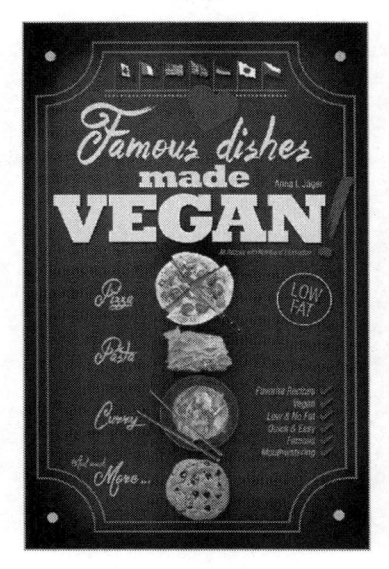

Your Favorite **Low-Fat Vegan** Cooking Recipes, Quick & Easy

If you think that following the vegan diet means that you can't enjoy delicious, flavorful, famous foods then think again! In this book of Low Fat Vegan Recipes you will find a collection of delectable vegan recipes that are low in fat but high in flavor. Enjoy some of your favorite dishes from around the world including pancakes, pizza, cupcakes, and more!

In addition to being low fat and vegan-friendly, these recipes are also high-carb and low (or no) fat, which makes them work for the *RawTill4* diet as well.

Simply put, this book gives you some of the fastest, easiest ways to enjoy your favorite foods while following the Vegan diet. If you are ready to transform your life and enjoy some delicious recipes, get this book!

ISBN-13: 978-1508858423
ISBN-10: 150885842X

Disclaimer

This book is intended as a reference volume only, not as a medical manual. Nothing written in this book should be viewed as a substitute for competent medical care. The information given here is designed to help you make more informed decisions about your health. It is not intended as a substitute for any treatment that may have been prescribed by your doctor. If you suspect that you have a medical problem, we urge you to seek competent medical help. Also, you should not undertake any changes in diet or exercise patterns without first consulting your physician, especially if you are currently being treated for any risk factor related to heart disease, high blood pressure or adult-onset diabetes. If you follow a low-fat vegan plan strictly for more than 3 years, or if you are pregnant and nursing, then consult your physician in regard to taking a minimum of 5 micrograms of supplemental vitamin B12 daily.

Neither the publisher nor the author disengaged in rendering professional advice or services to the individual reader. Neither the author nor the publisher shall be liable or responsible for any loss or damage allegedly arising from any information or suggestion in this book.

Mention of specific companies, organizations or authorities in this book does not imply endorsement by the publisher, nor does mention of specific companies, organizations, or authorities imply that they endorse the book. Further, the publisher does not have any control over and does not assume any responsibility for author or third-party websites or their content.

Copyright & Legal Information

Copyright © Anna I. Jäger

All rights reserved. No part of this publication may be reproduced or transmitted in any form or by any means, electronic or mechanical, including photocopying, recording, or any other information storage and retrieval system, without the written permission from the copyright owner except in the case of brief quotations or brief quotations embodied in critical articles or reviews.

„Reverse Diabetes Naturally;
A Guide to Effectively Lower Your Blood Sugar Without Drugs by Following the Right Diet"
by Jäger, Anna, I.;
Series: Diabetes Cure for Diabetics Type 2 (1)
Published by: Anna I. Jäger

First Edition February 2015

Co-Author: Lindsay Zortman, Debbie Alvarez

Image rights: © elenabsl

Updated January 23rd, 2016 (Version 2.0)

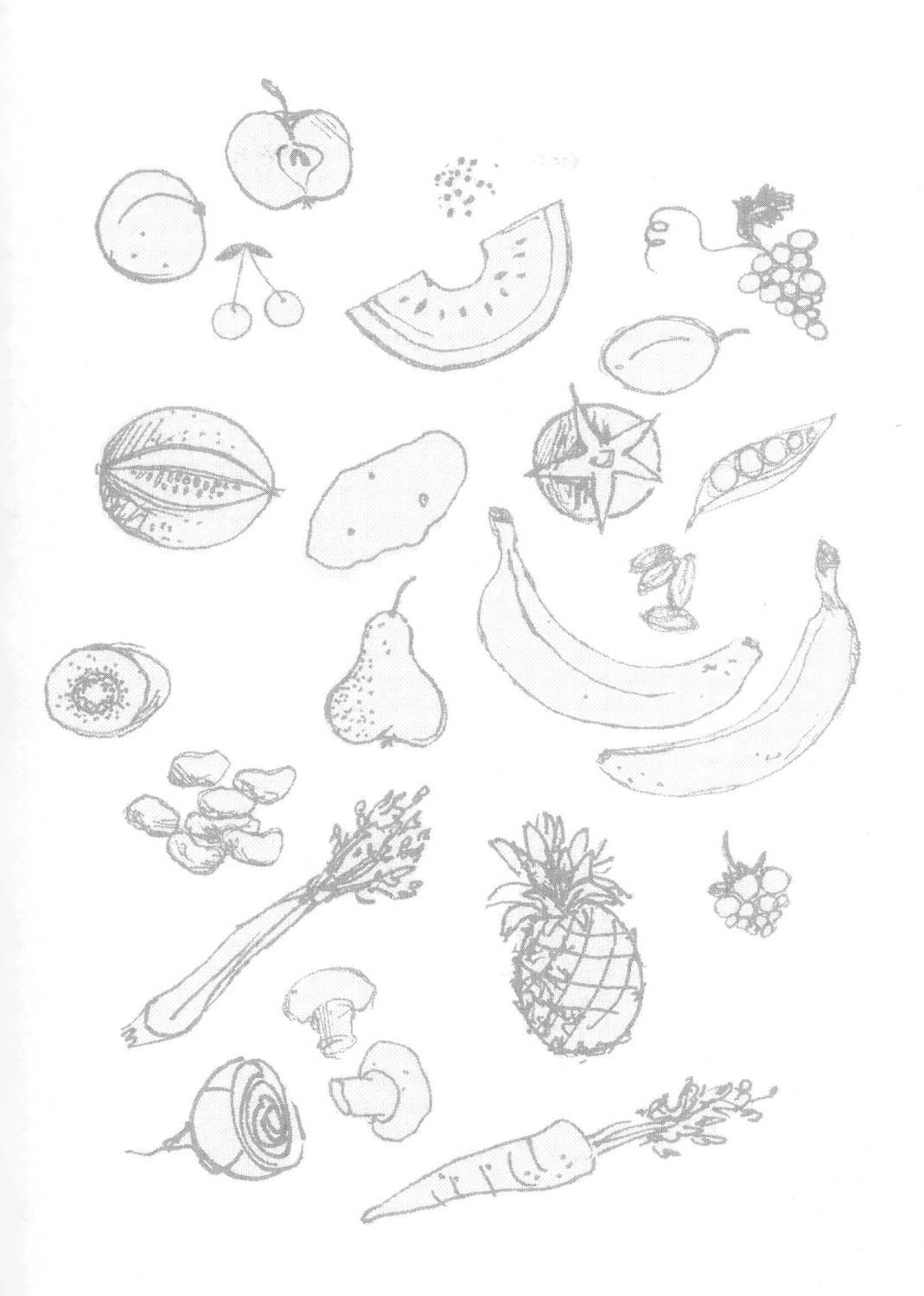

Made in the USA
Columbia, SC
01 March 2019